PHARMACOLOGY - RESEARCH, SAFETY TESTING AND REGULATION

CARBAMAZEPINE

INDICATIONS, CONTRAINDICATIONS AND ADVERSE EFFECTS

PHARMACOLOGY - RESEARCH, SAFETY TESTING AND REGULATION

Additional books in this series can be found on Nova's website under the Series tab.

Additional e-books in this series can be found on Nova's website under the eBooks tab.

PHARMACOLOGY - RESEARCH, SAFETY TESTING AND REGULATION

CARBAMAZEPINE

INDICATIONS, CONTRAINDICATIONS AND ADVERSE EFFECTS

BERNADETTE A. WOODS
EDITOR

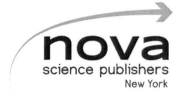

nova
science publishers
New York

Copyright © 2017 by Nova Science Publishers, Inc.

All rights reserved. No part of this book may be reproduced, stored in a retrieval system or transmitted in any form or by any means: electronic, electrostatic, magnetic, tape, mechanical photocopying, recording or otherwise without the written permission of the Publisher.

We have partnered with Copyright Clearance Center to make it easy for you to obtain permissions to reuse content from this publication. Simply navigate to this publication's page on Nova's website and locate the "Get Permission" button below the title description. This button is linked directly to the title's permission page on copyright.com. Alternatively, you can visit copyright.com and search by title, ISBN, or ISSN.

For further questions about using the service on copyright.com, please contact:
Copyright Clearance Center
Phone: +1-(978) 750-8400   Fax: +1-(978) 750-4470   E-mail: info@copyright.com.

NOTICE TO THE READER

The Publisher has taken reasonable care in the preparation of this book, but makes no expressed or implied warranty of any kind and assumes no responsibility for any errors or omissions. No liability is assumed for incidental or consequential damages in connection with or arising out of information contained in this book. The Publisher shall not be liable for any special, consequential, or exemplary damages resulting, in whole or in part, from the readers' use of, or reliance upon, this material. Any parts of this book based on government reports are so indicated and copyright is claimed for those parts to the extent applicable to compilations of such works.

Independent verification should be sought for any data, advice or recommendations contained in this book. In addition, no responsibility is assumed by the publisher for any injury and/or damage to persons or property arising from any methods, products, instructions, ideas or otherwise contained in this publication.

This publication is designed to provide accurate and authoritative information with regard to the subject matter covered herein. It is sold with the clear understanding that the Publisher is not engaged in rendering legal or any other professional services. If legal or any other expert assistance is required, the services of a competent person should be sought. FROM A DECLARATION OF PARTICIPANTS JOINTLY ADOPTED BY A COMMITTEE OF THE AMERICAN BAR ASSOCIATION AND A COMMITTEE OF PUBLISHERS.

Additional color graphics may be available in the e-book version of this book.

Library of Congress Cataloging-in-Publication Data

ISBN: 978-1-53611-954-1
Library of Congress Control Number: 2017940852

Published by Nova Science Publishers, Inc. † New York

CONTENTS

PREFACE

Carbamazepine (CBZ) is a member of the iminostilbene family, and it possesses a carbonyl group that is essential for its antiepileptic activity. It has been demonstrated and is widely accepted that CBZ is effective in the control of epileptic crises; unfortunately, there is scattered information concerning whether CBZ can aid in the sleep disorders produced by these crises. Chapter One evaluates the effect of the administration of CBZ on the sleep patterns in a model of epilepsy induced by KA and its pharmacokinetic and pharmacodynamic correlation. Chapter Two discusses the use of carbamazepine in freediving. Carbamazepine produces the protective effect of hypoxia and prolongs latency for the development of convulsions and death. Chapter Three is a review of current reports on the presence of carbamazepine in the environment, complemented with a general overview of typical (usually low) efficiencies with which conventional wastewater treatment plants are capable of removing carbamazepine from domestic wastewaters. CBZ is hardly biodegraded (the removal efficiency is <10%) through the conventional activated sludge process and the white-rot fungus (WRF) is reported the only microorganism to degrade it efficiently. The final chapter aims to enhance the removal performance of WRF reactor toward CBZ under non-sterile conditions during long-term operation.

Chapter 1 - CarBamaZepine (CBZ) is a member of the Iminostilbene family, and it possess a carbonyl group that is essential for its antiepileptic activity. It has been demonstrated and is widely accepted that CBZ is effective in the control of epileptic crises; unfortunately, there is scattered information concerning whether CBZ can aid in the sleep disorders produced by these crises. Because CBZ is one of the drugs that is most employed as an antiepileptic, it is important to analyze its effect on the electrical activity of the brain and sleep patterns under experimental and clinical conditions.

The main purpose of this study was to evaluate the effect of the administration of CBZ on the sleep patterns in a model of epilepsy induced by KA and its pharmacokinetic and pharmacodynamic correlation.

In this study, 40 male Wistar rats (weighing 250–280 g) were employed. Group 1 KA animals ($n = 10$) were chronically implanted with bipolar electrodes in the motor cortex, this to register cerebral activity (ElectroEncephaloGram [EEG]) and that of the neck muscles to obtain the muscular activity (ElectroMyoGram [EMG]). An electroencephalographic registry was taken from day 1 (Control); on day 2, Kainic Acid (KA) (10 mg/kg) was administered to induce the epileptic crisis and the registry continued for 5 additional days. Group 2 (CBZ+KA) animals ($n = 10$) followed the same chronic implantation of bipolar electrodes: day 1 (Control) was registered, and on Day 2, CBZ (25 mg/kg) was administered 30 min prior to the injection of KA, with the registry continuing for 3 additional days. Histological samples were obtained to evaluate the damage elicited by the drugs employed ($n = 10$). Group 3 animals ($n = 10$) were implanted with a cannula in the jugular vein to obtain the blood samples; a baseline sample was taken prior to the administration of CBZ (25 mg/kg), Subsequently, blood samples were taken at 10, 20, and 40 min and at 1, 2, 4, 8, 12, 24, 36, and 48 h for the pharmacokinetic analysis. To assess the differences between the pharmacokinetic and pharmacodynamic parameters, a Student t test for unpaired samples was performed, and $p < 0.05$ was considered to denote a significant difference. To evaluate the differences between the groups of EEG, the data was analyzed by a one-way ANalysis Of VAriance (ANOVA) (*$p < 0.01$ and **$p < 0.001$). The results showed a total absence of sleep during the first experimental day (Day 1) in Group 1 (KA), while in Group 2 (CBZ+KA), a partial recovery of Slow Wave Sleep (SWS) was also exhibited also during Day 1. Histological analysis revealed similar damage to that present in temporal-lobe epilepsy. The effect of CBZ was favorable, given that the crises significantly decreased when administered with CBZ, the latter demonstrated by comparison of the pharmacokinetics with the crisis.

Conclusion. CBZ significantly decreases crises; however, only partial recovery of sleep is present and the Rapid Eye Movement (REM) sleep is the most damaged. A correlation was present between the pharmacokinetic and pharmacodynamic profiles of CBZ and its effect exerted on the sleep-wake cycle.

Chapter 2 - Doping in sport has been known since the Olympic Games in ancient Greece. Doping allows less capable athletes to achieve superior results. In non-Olympic sports doping is still poorly controlled. There have been reports on the use of carbamazepine in freediving. Carbamazepine produces the protective effect of hypoxia and prolongs latency for the development of convulsions and death. The World Anti-Doping Agency (WADA) and all organizations responsible for freediving started prohibiting the use of doping and implementing continuous monitoring, and thus enabled this beautiful activity to become an Olympic sport.

Chapter 3 - Carbamazepine is a largely prescribed drug worldwide but in the latest years has also become notoriously known as a ubiquitous contaminant of aquatic environments. Indeed, the frequent detection of carbamazepine in effluents of wastewater treatment plants is due to the general inefficiency of conventional wastewater treatment processes to remove this recalcitrant contaminant from incoming contaminated wastewaters. Several studies confirmed that carbamazepine is persistent to bio and photodegradation in the aquatic media and, due to its recalcitrant behaviour, it has been proposed as a possible anthropogenic marker in the aquatic environment. However, up until now only scarce information has been collected in regard to the potential ecological impacts of carbamazepine. It is, thus, very important to consolidate the knowledge about its behaviour and fate in the environment and assess the risks it poses to aquatic ecosystems.

This work is a review of current reports on the presence of carbamazepine in the environment, complemented with a general overview of typical (usually low) efficiencies with which conventional wastewater treatment plants are capable of removing carbamazepine from domestic wastewaters. Furthermore, processes and influencing factors that determine the fate of carbamazepine in wastewater treatment plants and in the environment are presented and discussed. Finally, various technologies that have been under study and development over recent years in response to the general inefficiency of conventional wastewater treatment processes in treating carbamazapine and other emerging pollutants are outline and discussed briefly. Hopefully, prospects for significant improvements in carbamazepine removal efficiencies and potential means to achieve that goal in the future are pointed out in this work.

Chapter 4 - Carbamazepine (CBZ) is a pharmaceutically active compound that has been detected in many water bodies worldwide and is classified as a micropollutant. CBZ is hardly biodegraded (removal efficiency <10%) through the conventional activated sludge process and the white-rot fungus

(WRF) is reported the only microorganism to degrade it efficiently. Even though the WRF reactor has been applied to remove CBZ from wastewater, the performances varied considerably. In addition, it is still difficult to maintain a stable long-term reactor performance due to the bacterial contamination. This study aims to enhance the removal performance of WRF reactor toward CBZ under non-sterile conditions during long-term operation. The possibility of a WRF strain *Phanerochaete chrysosporium* immobilized on wooden chips to remove CBZ under non-sterile conditions was investigated. The CBZ removal efficiency in artificially contaminated water was improved around 30% in 7 days when the fungal immobilization was used. Adsorption was the main contributor to the CBZ removal at the early stage. However, bioremoval was considered the main removal mechanism afterwards. A countercurrent seepage bioreactor with *P. chrysosporium* immobilized on wooden chips was developed and continuously fed with synthetic domestic wastewater spiked with CBZ (1,000 μg/L) under non-sterile conditions for 165 days. The average removal efficiency for CBZ reached $78.28 \pm 5.77\%$. The countercurrent seepage mode bioreactor proved to be conducive to increase the fungal resistance to the contamination by indigenous bacteria. The performance of CBZ removal was also evaluated under different reactor configuration consisted of a rotating suspension cartridge reactor immobilized with *P. chrysosporium* on polyurethane foam cubes. The reactor was continuously operated under non-sterile conditions for 160 days. The removal efficiency for CBZ exceeded 90% after one month of fungal adaptation by applying the intermittent operation mode and the progressive cut of external carbon source feeding. The CBZ removal mainly occurred biologically and adsorption accounted for only 7.7%. The bacterial contamination was suppressed effectively under non-sterile conditions for both reactor configurations considered as promising alternatives for the CBZ treatment in contaminated water.

In: Carbamazepine
Editor: Bernadette A. Woods

ISBN: 978-1-53611-954-1
© 2017 Nova Science Publishers, Inc.

Chapter 1

Neuroprotective Effect of Carbamazepine on the Sleep-Wake Cycle on a Model of Epilepsy Induced by Kainic Acid and Its Pharmacokinetic and Pharmacodynamic Correlation

Alfonso Alfaro-Rodríguez[1,]*, PhD,
Samuel Reyes-Long[1], MD,
José Luis Cortes-Altamirano[2], PhD,
Adriana Olmos-Hernández[1], PhD,
Rebeca Uribe-Escamilla[1], PhD,
Angélica González-Maciel[3], PhD
and Cindy Bandala[1], PhD

[1]Department of Neuroscience, National Institute of Rehabilitation,
Mexico City, Mexico
[2]Department of Biological and Health Sciences, Universidad Autónoma
Metropolitana, Mexico City, Mexico
[3]Laboratory of Cell and Tissue Morphology,
National Institute of Pediatrics, Mexico City, Mexico

---

* Corresponding author: E-mail: alfa1360@yahoo.com.mx.

Abstract

CarBamaZepine (CBZ) is a member of the Iminostilbene family, and it possess a carbonyl group that is essential for its antiepileptic activity. It has been demonstrated and is widely accepted that CBZ is effective in the control of epileptic crises; unfortunately, there is scattered information concerning whether CBZ can aid in the sleep disorders produced by these crises. Because CBZ is one of the drugs that is most employed as an antiepileptic, it is important to analyze its effect on the electrical activity of the brain and sleep patterns under experimental and clinical conditions.

The main purpose of this study was to evaluate the effect of the administration of CBZ on the sleep patterns in a model of epilepsy induced by KA and its pharmacokinetic and pharmacodynamic correlation.

In this study, 40 male Wistar rats (weighing 250–280 g) were employed. Group 1 KA animals ($n = 10$) were chronically implanted with bipolar electrodes in the motor cortex, this to register cerebral activity (ElectroEncephaloGram [EEG]) and that of the neck muscles to obtain the muscular activity (ElectroMyoGram [EMG]). An electroencephalographic registry was taken from day 1 (Control); on day 2, Kainic Acid (KA) (10 mg/kg) was administered to induce the epileptic crisis and the registry continued for 5 additional days. Group 2 (CBZ+KA) animals ($n = 10$) followed the same chronic implantation of bipolar electrodes: day 1 (Control) was registered, and on Day 2, CBZ (25 mg/kg) was administered 30 min prior to the injection of KA, with the registry continuing for 3 additional days. Histological samples were obtained to evaluate the damage elicited by the drugs employed ($n = 10$). Group 3 animals ($n = 10$) were implanted with a cannula in the jugular vein to obtain the blood samples; a baseline sample was taken prior to the administration of CBZ (25 mg/kg), Subsequently, blood samples were taken at 10, 20, and 40 min and at 1, 2, 4, 8, 12, 24, 36, and 48 h for the pharmacokinetic analysis. To assess the differences between the pharmacokinetic and pharmacodynamic parameters, a Student t test for unpaired samples was performed, and $p < 0.05$ was considered to denote a significant difference. To evaluate the differences between the groups of EEG, the data was analyzed by a one-way ANalysis Of VAriance (ANOVA) (*$p < 0.01$ and **$p < 0.001$). The results showed a total absence of sleep during the first experimental day (Day 1) in Group 1 (KA), while in Group 2 (CBZ+KA), a partial recovery of Slow Wave Sleep (SWS) was also exhibited also during Day 1. Histological analysis revealed similar damage to that present in temporal-lobe epilepsy. The effect of CBZ was favorable, given that the crises significantly decreased when administered with CBZ, the latter demonstrated by comparison of the pharmacokinetics with the crisis.

Conclusion. CBZ significantly decreases crises; however, only partial recovery of sleep is present and the Rapid Eye Movement (REM) sleep is the most damaged. A correlation was present between the pharmacokinetic and pharmacodynamic profiles of CBZ and its effect exerted on the sleep-wake cycle.

INTRODUCTION

Kainic Acid (KA) is one of the most employed pharmaceutical in animal models of epilepsy. This model has been proposed due to its potency in the induction of a syndrome characterized by limbic acute status epilepticus and subsequent neuronal damage, similar to that presented in temporal lobe epilepsy in humans.

CarbaMaZepine (CBZ) is a member of the Iminostilbene family and it possess a carbonyl group that is essential for its antiepileptic activity. It presents a chemical relationship with tricyclic antidepressant drugs, and its tricyclic structure is what renders it insoluble in water (Figure 1). CBZ is a first-line option for the treatment of seizure disorders (partial seizures, generalized tonic-clonic seizures) and is among the most frequently used AntiEpileptic Drugs (AED) in combination therapy [1]. CBZ can also be utilized in the treatment of attention deficit and hyperactivity disorders, schizophrenia, phantom limb syndrome, complex regional pain syndrome, and post-traumatic stress disorder [2, 3].

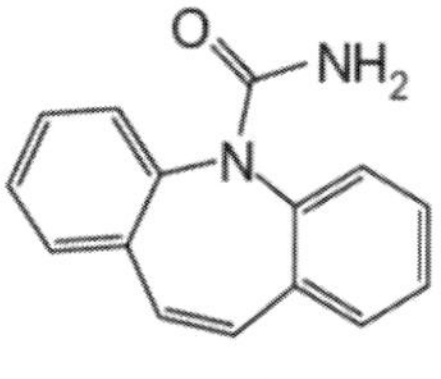

Figure 1. Structural formula of Carbamazepine.

Carbamazepine in Epilepsy

It has been previously described in animal and human studies that CBZ exerts action on the voltage-gated Na+ channels; additionally, it increases the frequency of noradrenergic neurons discharges on the Locus Coeruleus of rats [4]. CBZ stabilizes the hyperexcited neuronal membranes, inhibiting repetitive neuronal discharges and reducing the synaptic propagation of excitatory pulses. It is possible that the blockade of voltage-gated Na+ channels comprises the main mechanism of action [5]. There are two main ways in which CBZ can attenuate an epileptic crisis: reduction of the excessive discharge of pathologically altered neurons and limitation of excitation from the focus, and prevention of detonation and interruption of the normal neuron group.

It has been demonstrated and is widely accepted that CBZ is effective in the control of epileptic crises; unfortunately, there is scattered information concerning whether CBZ can aid in the sleep disorders produced by these crises.

Epilepsy and Sleep Disorders

Two of the most frequent complaints of patients with epilepsy include disturbed sleep and excessive daytime drowsiness [6]. The symptoms can be explained by the broad relationship between nictemeral organization of the sleep-vigilance (wakefulness) cycle and the incidence of epileptic crises [7, 8, 9]. In humans and animals, sleep patterns can be disturbed by epileptic attacks, an effect that depends on the magnitude of the seizures [10, 11]. Sleep can exert a strong influence on both seizure activation and interictal ElectroEncephaloGram (EEG) abnormalities [12, 13]; for example, it has been shown that sleep patterns respond differently to different types of crisis [14].

Sleep eases temporal lobe epilepsy; hence, epilepsy that originates in this region of the brain is considered as nocturnal seizures [9, 15, 16]. The relationship between epilepsy and the phasic events of sleep has been studied in patients who have exhibited either focal or generalized seizures and in animal models of temporal lobe epilepsy of humans [17].

In contrast, Ng & Bianchi [18] conducted a retrospective study in which they compared self-reported disturbances in sleep architecture among patients with epilepsy, patients with insomnia undergoing polysomnography, and patients with obstructive sleep apnea. The authors found that sleep misperception occurs similarly in patients with epilepsy and in patients without epilepsy with insomnia.

Despite the numerous studies mentioned previously that have related epileptic crises with sleep, there are few reports describing the possible influence exerted by this crisis on the organization of sleep.

In the temporal-lobe epilepsy model employed herein, significant disorganization was demonstrated of the sleep-vigilance (wakefulness) cycle, involving Slow Wave Sleep (SWS) and Rapid Eye Movement (REM) sleep.

Several neurotransmitters are associated with the firing and maintaining of sleep. Several studies indicate that Serotonin (5-HT) is involved in the regulation of functions such as memory, learning, sleep, and pain [19, 20, 21], In addition, neurophysiological data has shown that neurons in the Dorsal Raphe Nucleus (DRN) fire at their maximal during vigilance (wakefulness) and that its activity diminishes during sleep, reaching minimal levels during REM sleep [22, 23]. The DRN has been related with the establishment of SWS [24], while REM sleep depends on the serotoninergic activity present during vigilance (wakefulness) and promotes the formation of hypothalamic peptides where the mechanisms of REM sleep are integrated.

With regard to REM sleep, it is noteworthy that in the pons of the brainstem, several cellular nuclei are located that generate its different components, such as the Locus Coeruleus (LC), the principal producer of NorAdrenaline (NA) at the pons levels. NA produces hyperpolarization of motoneurons and with the latter, inhibition of muscular tone [25]. In accordance with the Hobson & McCarley model of reciprocal interaction [26, 27], the presence of the sleep states is controlled by two groups of neurons that are located in the reticular formation of the brainstem: REM-on neurons, which are located in the LateroDorsal Tegmental (LDT) nucleus and in the PenduncaloPonTine (PPT) nucleus, and REM-off neurons, monoaminergic cell groups including the 5-HT and NA, the former deriving mainly from the DRN and the latter, from the LC [28–25]. Evidence of this hypothesis originates from the knowledge that Acetylcholine (ACh) plays an essential role in the foundation of REM sleep. It has been shown that the main structures in charge of the firing and maintenance of REM sleep are located in the PPT and the LDT [29].

Carbamazepine and Sleep Disorders

It has been clinically and experimentally reported that CBZ is a very effective drug against psychomotor disorders and grand mal seizures [30]. Because CBZ is one of the drugs most frequently employed as an antiepileptic, it is important to analyze its effect on electrical activity and sleep patterns, in a model of epilepsy triggered by the administration of KA. The anticonvulsant activity of CBZ has been demonstrated in crises chemically or electrically induced in rats and mice.

Several studies have focused in the membrane permeability point at which CBZ diminishes the flow of sodium (Na) and calcium (Ca2$^+$) [31] and, in a lesser amount, potassium (K). CBZ also inhibits the uptake and release of Norepinephrine (Ne) from cerebral synaptosomes [32]. Also, data obtained from slices of the brain suggest that CBZ action is independent of the GABAergic system, in that CBZ does not influence the uptake of Gamma AminoButyric Acid (GABA) [33]. Controversial data exist with respect to the post-tetanic potentiation exerted by CBZ [34].

Antiepileptic drugs can be identified in several experimental models and their capacity to abolish epileptic crises can be tested. These models have provided tools for clarifying the mechanism of action of different drugs in the regulation of the epileptogenesis.

Due to the similar structure of Glutamate (Glu) and KA, the latter is considered a powerful neuroexcitatory and neurotoxic substance acting on the Central Nervous System (CNS) of mammals [35, 36]. The principal quality that renders KA relevant for the research of epilepsy is that it induces a syndrome characterized by acute limbic status epilepticus with subsequent neuronal damage, similar to that presented in temporal-lobe epilepsy in humans [37]. Thus, its administration induces a model similar to this type of epilepsy [38].

The administration of KA is mainly systemic, because it presents the same behavioral and neuropathological changes found when administered locally in the brain [39]. Through this administration route, mechanical and high concentration- related damages are avoided [38].

Given that the brain's electrical activity is very sensitive to the intake of drugs, the purpose of this study was to determine the efficacy with which CBZ diminishes the epileptiform patterns produced by the administration of KA and, at the same time, increases the threshold required to trigger convulsive crises.

Due to the fact that clinically, CBZ is one of the most employed drugs against epileptic seizures, it is important to assess the pharmacological effect of CBZ on the brain's electrical activity, mainly in sleep wake-pattern sleep. Additionally, it is relevant to evaluate the neuromorphological alterations produced by KA-induced status epilepticus as a valid model of temporal lobe-epilepsy and the prior administration of CBZ. The KA model, among others, has allowed the study of several anticonvulsant drugs and their effects.

METHODS

Forty male Wistar rats (weighing 250–280 g) were used. They were maintained under controlled conditions at a temperature of 25°C, relative humidity of 40% and photoperiodicity of 12-h light-dark cycle, with lights on at 8:00 h. The animals were fed a standard diet and drank water ad libitum. The animals were treated according to the Guide for the Care and Use of Experimental Animals [40] and under Official Mexican Standard NOM-062-ZOO-1999 [41]. All procedures were approved by the Research Ethics Committee of National Rehabilitation Institute (INR) "Luis Guillermo Ibarra Ibarra."

After a 7-day adjustment period in a soundproofed recording chamber where the polysomnographic studies were carried out, the rats were anesthetized with sodium pentobarbital (50 mg/kg intraperitoneally [i.p.]). After 5 min of the drug injection, the degree of sensitivity was tested by squeezing the last one third of the rat's tail until the rat reached the level of surgical anesthesia. After shaving and washing the incision area (frontal bone to occipital bone), the rats were placed on stereotaxic equipment (Stoelting Co., Wood Dale, IL, USA) and their body temperature was monitored and regulated with equipment for rats (CMA/150 temperature controller). After this, an iodine antiseptic solution was applied to the incision area and the incision was made with a #15 scalpel to obtain one craniocaudal cut. A skin incision ~1.0 cm in length was made at the level of the frontal and occipital bone. Once the skull was exposed, a suture was placed in the skull according to the pre-established coordinates and the animals were implanted with a stainless steel bipolar electrode on the sensorimotor cortex for EEG recording. Two additional stainless steel electrodes were placed on the neck muscles for ElectroMyoGram (EMG) recording. The incision was then sutured with non-absorbable 2-0 nylon with a striated longitudinal body needle (SC-26) (26 mm, 3/8 reverse-circle cutting point). During the incision and suture, Lidocaine 10% was applied (each 100 g contained 10 g of Lidocaine base) with an atomizer (each pulsation of the valve releases 10 mg). Furazolidone with an atomizer was finally applied for 7 days (each 100 g contained 7.5 g Furazolidone). The animals recovered from surgery for 7 days. Seven days after post-operative recovery, the rats were placed in the soundproofed recording chamber for the polygraph recording and were given free access to food and water under controlled light–dark conditions (08:00–20:00 h light, 20:00–08:00 h dark) without movement restrictions. After becoming acclimated to the conditions described previously, the recordings were made.

The analysis of the EEG recording was carried out with a VIASYS Viking Quest Nicolet polygraph, which continuously recorded for 48 h. To integrate the different states of wakefulness, an MFPE device was employed (model 110).

The rats were allocated into two groups. The first of these was G1: the KA group (n = 10). Animals in this group underwent a Control polygraphic recording (EEG and EMG) during 10 h (on day 0) from 8:00 h to 18:00 h. Day 1 (experimental) KA (10 mg/kg, subcutaneously [sc]) was administered according to Sperk (1994), unleashing the epileptic crisis 30 min after the administration, and a 10-h polygraphic recording was performed to assess the effect of the KA. From day 2 (recovery) until day 5, three 10-h polygraphic recordings were performed (8:00–18:00 h), in order to observe the recovery of the different phases of the sleep-wake cycle. In the second group G2, the CBZ+AK group (n = 10), the animals also underwent a control polygraphic recording during 10 h (day 0) from 8:00 h to 18:00 h. On day 1 (experimental), the animals were administered CBZ (25 mg/kg of body weight, i.p., dissolved in ethanol and carboxymethylcellulose at 5%) through a gastric probe 30 min prior to the epileptic crisis induced by the administration of KA (10 mg/kg). Promptly, a 10-h polygraphic recording was performed and, at the same time, the intensity and duration of the convulsive crisis was quantified. From day 2 (recovery) until day 5, three 10-h polygraph recordings were carried out (8:00 h to 18:00 h), this to monitor any other effect of the convulsive crisis.

Histology

Subsequently, histological samples from a Control group (n = 10), and G1, G2, and G3 (administered CBZ 25 mg/kg) were obtained to evaluate the damage elicited by the drugs employed.

Under general anesthesia with pentobarbital (50 mg/kg), the rats were perfused via vascular system with saline solution and formalin buffered solution (ph 7.2). Brains were dissected and coronal slices were obtained (11 µm) for processing by means of the Cresyl Violet and Klüver–Barrera techniques.

Pharmacokinetics

In order to correlate between the epileptic crises and the pharmacokinetics of CBZ, G4 (n = 10) underwent surgery. Under general anesthesia with Ketamine (35 mg/kg) and Xylazine (3 mg/kg), the animals were implanted with a PolyEthylene (PE-10) cannula in the jugular vein for blood sampling and the pharmacokinetics of CBZ. Immediately after the surgical procedure, a baseline sample was taken; then, CBZ (25 mg/kg of body weight, i.p., dissolved in ethanol and carboxymethylcellulose at 5%) was administered. After this, 500-µL samples were taken at 10, 20, and 40 min and at 1, 2, 4, 8, 12, 24, and 48 h.

Identification of Carbamazepine in Plasma

The first solution was prepared dissolving CBZ and the internal standard (Oxcarbazepine) in methanol, reaching a concentration of 1 mg/ml. From this solution, dilutions from the mobile phase were conducted.

Chromatographic system: A Waters chromatograph was used, which consisted of a 510 pump, a U6-K injector, an inverse phase column, µBondapak C18, 3 cm in length, 3.9 mm in diameter, and with a 10-µm particle size, all connected to an UltraViolet (UV) detector with variable wavelength. The mobile phase consisted of a mixture of acetonitrile–water (30:70%, v/v) pumped at a 2-ml/min flow rate. Retention time for CBZ was 4.96 min and for the internal standard, this was 3.47 min (Oxcarbazepine).

Extraction method: Each plasma sample was put through an extraction method prior to its chromatographic analysis. This process consisted adding, to the 500 µl of blood plasma, 100 µl of CBZ with one of the concentrations of the curve (0.5, 1, 2, 5, and 10 µl/ml), and 100 µl of the internal standard (Oxcarbazepine) at a concentration of 10 µg/ml. Afterward, 4 ml of dichloromethane was added to each sample. This solution was mixed at high speed in the vortex for 2 min; next, the samples were centrifuged for 20 min at 3,500 rpm. The aqueous layer was aspirated and the organic phase was transferred into a clean test tube and evaporated to dryness utilizing a nitrogen evaporator at 45°C. The sample was then reconstituted with 200 µl mobile phase and 100 µl was injected to the chromatographic system. All determinations were performed at room temperature with a 215-nm wavelength.

EEG Data Analysis

The sleep analysis of each of the printed polygraphic recordings was analyzed visually according to Alfaro-Rodríguez and Gonzalez-Pina [42]. Briefly, they were classified as follows: Wakefulness (W), which was characterized by desynchronization of the EEG and the presence of muscle tone (EMG) that was accentuated during movements; Slow Wave Sleep (SWS), which was characterized by the presence of sleep spindles (slow waves with voltage >75V), and a decrease in EMG voltage, and during Paradoxical Sleep (PS), characterized by desynchronization of the EEG and an absence of EMG voltage. Mean values (mean ± Standard Error of the Mean [SEM]) were compared using a one-way Analysis Of VAriance (ANOVA), and subsequent comparisons between the groups were performed utilizing a Tukey test, *with* $p \leq 0.01$.

RESULTS

Under control conditions, G1 (KA 10 mg/kg) presented all three sleep phases (REM, SWS, and W). During wakefulness, animals presented different types of behavior as follows: exploring; feeding; drinking, and grooming. Cerebral activity was characterized by high-frequency wave patterns and low voltage patterns. EMG demonstrated electrical activity originating from the neck muscles; these muscles presented an increase in muscular tone.

During sleep, the conduct exhibited was that of pacific behavior as follows: the rats remained without activity during SWS; closed eyes without eye movement, with cerebral activity showing low-frequency wave patterns and high-voltage patterns; muscular tone decreased but the EMG was present; REM sleep followed SWS, EEG was similar to that observed during W, although muscular activity remained absent, with the exception of sporadic shakes in the extremities of the rat (Myoclonus).

Under control conditions, from 10 h of registry, rats remained in W for 182.72 ± 27.8 min, in SWS for 412.41 ± 29 min, and in REM, for 70.5 ± 8.3 min. Total time spent by the animals sleeping corresponded to 68%, of which 9% was REM sleep and 59% SWS. REM sleep presented only after SWS, never after W.

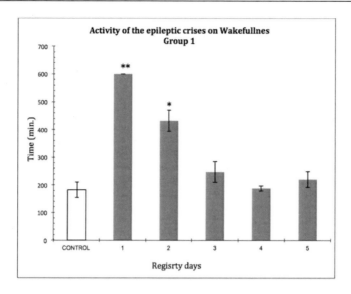

Figure 2. Animals underwent a registration period of 10 h. On day 1 KA was administered and animals remain in W the total period of registry (10 h). The time spent in W decreased through day 2 until day 5 ($n = 10$, SEM ± std *$p < 0.01$; **$p < 0.001$).

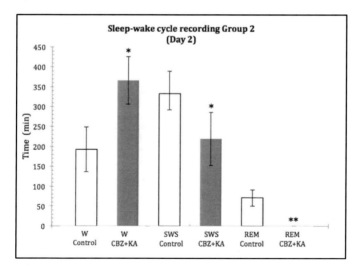

Figure 3. Sleep-wake cycle phases of Group 2 (CBZ + KA). White bars depict Control levels and grey bars experimental levels. The absence of REM sleep is to be noted. Wakefulness (W), Slow Wave Sleep (SWS), Rapid Eye Movement sleep (REM). ($n = 10$, SEM ± std *$p < 0.01$; **$p < 0.001$).

KA progressively induced the following motor alterations: tilting of the head; chewing activity, and shaking of the body and head ("wet dog" shakes). Next, the generalized crisis appeared, this conduct accompanied by intense salivation. For several hours, the animals presented recurring discharges until these decreased by the end of the registry period; the animals remained in W during the entire registry period and the latter caused the animals to become exhausted. Both SWS and REM sleep remained totally absent (Figure 2). On day 2, a recovery of SWS appeared (Figure 3), but it was not until day 4 day that SWS returned to its normal levels and, at the same time, W decreased progressively (Figure 2).

Effect of CBZ + KA on Sleep Patterns

Data showed that the epileptic crisis induced by the administration of KA affected the organization of sleep patterns.

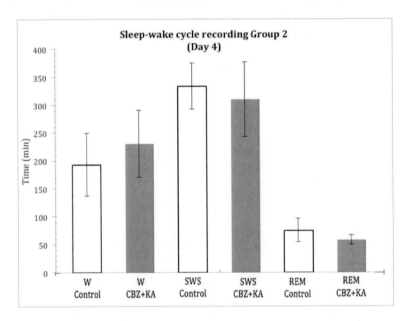

Figure 4. Sleep-wake cycle phases of Group 2 (CBZ + KA). White bars depict Control levels and grey bars experimental levels. Wakefulness (W), Slow Wave Sleep (SWS), Rapid Eye Movement sleep (REM). (n = 10, SEM ± std *p < 0.01; **p < 0.001).

On the other hand, CBZ (20 mg/kg) exerted a recovery effect on the sleep patterns when administered before KA. On day 1, SWS was present but with a decrease of 28% with regard to the control and with an increase of W of 28% with respect to control. The epileptic crisis decreased starting from hours 3 and 4. Both EEG and EMG showed notable differences when compared with G1 (Figure 2).

REM sleep remained inhibited during day 1 and through day 3 (Figure 3.), reaching control levels on day 4. Also on day 4, W reached its normal levels and SWS increased, but without reaching normal levels (Figure 4). It is noteworthy that in G2, the compensatory increase of REM sleep was also not present.

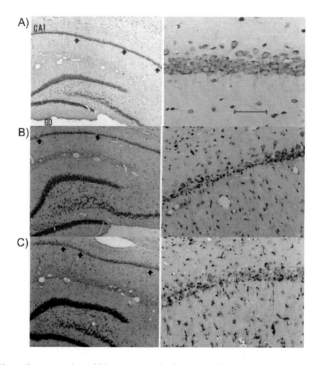

Figure 5. Microphotographs of hippocampal slices. A) Control B) KA and C) CBZ + KA. Black arrows show the regions of CA1 where the lesion and death of pyramidal neurons caused by KA was found (left). A close up of the areas damaged is shown (right). In the Control group an even column of pyramidal neurons is present, in the same area of experimental groups some pyramidal neurons are present (black arrows) but also some remains of dead neurons (overstained points). Above and below the column of the pyramidal neuron column extended hyperchromatin remains are present, belonging to neuronal processes. Cresyl violet staining technique. Bar scale = 10 μm.

HISTOLOGICAL ANALYSIS

In the control group, a normal morphology of neurons was found in hippocampus and cerebellum (Figures 5 and 6), with similar conditions were found in G3 (CBZ).

G1 (KA) animals presented a selective lesion in areas CA1 and CA3, and in the cingulate gyrus of the hippocampus: after the death of neurons, a discontinuity appeared in the cortical plate of pyramidal neurons in CA1, and necrosis in groups of pyramidal neurons (Figure 5). In the cerebellum, Purkinje neurons were affected, and necrosis was also found in great numbers of these cells (Figure 6).

G2 (CBZ + KA) presented the same lesion in pyramidal neurons of CA1 as described previously, although in a larger area than that of the G1 (Figure 5). In G2, we also found that in dentate gyrus, medial thalamus, and piriform cortex, neuronal death and neutrophil damage were both present (Figure 6).

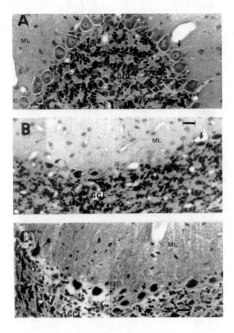

Figure 6. Sagittal slices of rat brains. A) Control B) Group 1 (KA) C) Group 2 (CBZ + KA). In B remains of Purkinje cells are all that remains in the area corresponding to them (Black arrows). In C necrotic remains of Purkinje cells and extensive zones with damages in neuropil of the molecular layer (ML) and in the granule cell layer were present. Bar scale = 5 μm.

PHARMACOKINETICS

Validation of the CBZ Quantification Method

Linearity of the method was obtained by analyzing blood plasma samples containing a standard solution of drugs at concentration ranges of 0.22–5 µl/ml according to pilot tests. Five points were chosen (0.22, 0.50, 1, 2, and 5 µl/ml) and five determinations were made for each point. Quantification was carried out by the internal standard method; the relation between CBZ heights and the internal standard was measured.

For preparation of the stock solution, we began with standard solutions of CBZ at a 1-mg/ml concentration dissolved in chromatography-grade ethanol. From these, the solutions required for the calibration curve were prepared by means of dilutions with mobile phase, in the previously mentioned range.

Calibration Curves

To obtain calibration, we employed a 100-µl blood sample with 60 µl/ml from the internal standard for each CBZ concentration (0.22, 0.50, 1, 2, and 5 µl/ml).

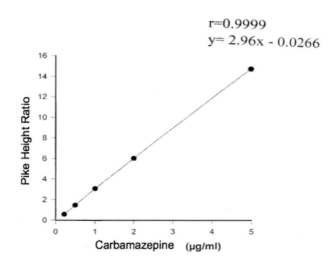

Figure 7. Calibration curve of CBZ. Pike Height Ratio is the coefficient of the chromatographic pikes height of CBZ over the internal standard Each point represents means (± S.E.) of eight determinations.

Figure 7 depicts the relation of the spikes (height of the spike of CBZ/height of the internal standard) according to the blood concentration of CBZ and also, the equation of the line adjusting experimental data with a high correlation.

Table 1 show that the coefficient of variation (CV) is less than 9.40%, which indicated that the method employed is adequate for the determination of CBZ in rat's blood. The limit of quantification of the method was 0.22 μL/mL.

Table 1. Coefficient of variation and accuracy of the method employed for the determination of CBZ in blood. Data is expressed as SEM ± std

Nominal Concentration (μg/ml)	Mean Concentration (μg/ml)	Accuracy as RD (%)	Precision as CV (%)
0.22	0.20 ± 0.008	90.91	9.40
0.50	0.5026 ± 0.016	101.12	7.99
1	1.05 ± 0.033	105	7.81
2	2.04 ±0.071	102	8.59
5	5.00 ± 0.087	100	4.28

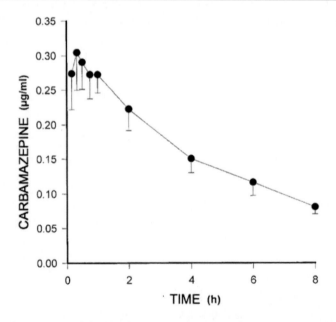

Figure 8. Time courses of the blood concentration of CBZ. Each point represents means (± S.E.) of six determinations.

Figure 8 shows the pharmacokinetic of CBZ (25 mg/kg) in which means (± S.E.) of the time courses from blood concentrations expressed as µg/ml function of time. The kinetic of CBZ suffers an abrupt fall for then to ascend gradually. From the time courses, the pharmacokinetic parameters were obtained, these comprehend by the area under the curve (AUC).

From each individual graphic, C_{max} and t_{max} were obtained. The Area Under the Curve (AUC) was calculated by means of the trapezoidal method (Rowland & Tozer, 1989) until the last simple point. Pharmacokinetic parameters were calculated independently according to Gibaldi [43].

DISCUSSION

The data showed that during the acute state of the administration of KA, sleep patterns were heavily altered; the animals remained in a state of vigilance (wakefulness) and the first symptoms of convulsive crisis appeared. SWS and REM sleep were completely abolished during a relatively long time period. The effects caused by KA in this study were similar to those present in previous studies [44, 45, 46]. The results also are very similar to those reported in temporal lobe epilepsy in humans [38].

It is known that KA exerts an excitatory effect on the kainite receptors [47, 48] and during KA acute administration; Glu is released over the hippocampus [49, 50]. Also, heavily decreased levels of the Glutamate decarboxylase, an enzyme that catalyzes the formation of GABA from Glu, have been found in different brain areas: amygdala; piriform cortex; lateral septum, and hippocampus. All of these observations support the hypothesis that epilepsy may be related with malfunctioning in the GABAergic system [51]. This may in part explain the negative effects caused by KA-induced epileptic crisis on the sleep patterns, because GABA plays a crucial role in the regulation of the sleep-vigilance (wakefulness) cycle.

In particular, stimulation of the $GABA_A$ receptor increases the time employed in sleep [52]. Despite that disorganization of the sleep pattern may be involved with the incidence of the epileptic crisis, the origin of these changes are not clear.

The LC is related with the regulation of REM sleep; when destroyed, this gives rise to a decrease in this sleep phase and also increases the susceptibility of epileptic crises. It is probable that KA may cause a transitory inhibition of the LC, because a relation between the LC and hippocampal structures have been observed, and additionally, it can act as a modulator of hippocampus during REM sleep [53]. These arguments favor the relationships between the incidence of epileptic crises and the decrease of REM sleep.

Crises triggered by KA have been related with the inhibition of SWS and REM sleep. However, the decrease of REM sleep may be eased by the recurrence of these crises and by generalized crises. These findings partially agree with those of the sleep recordings of patients immediately after a generalized crisis, in which they presented a transitory decrease in REM sleep [7, 12]. A similar decrease has been described in other temporal lobe epilepsy models, where the epileptic activity was caused by electrical stimulations applied on the amygdala or the hippocampus [54, 55]. A decrease in REM sleep was observed, although after electrical stimulation, it returned to its normal levels. Similar finding were present in this study, given that the sleep inhibitions persisted, but only for 3 days; after that, all behavioral and electrographic alterations disappeared. This suggests that inhibition of sleep and a long period of insomnia are not only caused by the physiological intervention of drugs or electrical stimulation, but also by the neurophysiological mechanisms that regulate the sleep-wake cycle, such as the medial pontine reticular formation. It is interesting that a compensation of sleep is not present when decreasing the different sleep phases, as observed when sleep deprivation is caused by other means [56].

The literature describes that CBZ presents a protector effect. There is evidence in animal models that Na-channel antagonists prevent the neuronal damage caused by local or general ischemia [57]. *In vivo* studies have demonstrated that some drugs, including CBZ, reduce the rodent's brain damage after focal ischemia [58, 59, 60]. Also, CBZ protects cortical cultures from Veratridine-induced cell death at a 10-μM dose [61]; also, this particular study suggested that other mechanisms, such as Na-channel antagonism, may be involved in the neuroprotective effect.

CBZ diminishes the severity of the convulsive crisis, favoring recovery of SWS, even though REM sleep remains inhibited; thus, only a partial recovery of sleep is observed. A compensatory rebound of REM sleep was not present. There was a correlation between the pharmacokinetic and pharmacodynamic profiles of CBZ and its effect exerted on the sleep-wake cycle.

REFERENCES

[1] Stokis, A., Chanteaux, H., Rosa, H., Rolan, P. (2015). Brivaracetam and carbamazepine interaction in healthy subjects and *in vitro*. *Epilepsy Research.* 113:19-17.

[2] Niederhofer, H. (2011). Combining Carbamazepine, neuroleptics and acetylcholinesterase inhibitors with Methylphenidate only reduces adverse side effects, but is less effective than a combination with Atomoxetine. *Correspondence/Medical Hypotheses.* 17:761-767.

[3] Rogawski, M. A. & Löscher, W. (2004). The neurobiology of antiepileptic drugs for the treatment of nonepileptic conditions. *Nature Medicine.* 10(7):685-692.

[4] Alrashood, S. T. (2016). Carbamazepine. In: *Profiles of Drug Substances, Excipients, and Related Methodology* Vol 41. Elsevier Inc.

[5] Okada, M., Kiryu, K., Kawata, Y. (1997). Determination of the effects of caffeine and carbamazepine on striatal dopamine release by microdyalisis. *European Journal of Pharmacology.* 32:181-188.

[6] Legros, B. & Bazil C. W. (2003). Effects of antiepileptic drugs on sleep architecture: a pilot study. *Sleep Medicine.* 4:51-55.

[7] Bazil, C.W., Castro, L.H., Walczakt, T.S. (2000). Reduction of rapid eye movement sleep by diurnal and nocturnal seizures in temporal lobe epilepsy. *Archives of Neurolology.* 57:363-368.

[8] McNamara, J. O. & Shin, C. (1994). Mechanism of epilepsy. *Annual Reviews on Medicine.* 45:379-389.

[9] Malow, B., Selwa, L., Ross, D., Aldrich, M. (1999). Lateralizing value of interictal spikes on overnight sleep-EEG studies in Temporal Lobe Epilepsy. *Epilepsia.* 40(11):1597-1592.

[10] Gigli, G. L., Placidini, F., Diomedi, M., Maschio, M., Silvestre, G., Scalise, A., Marciani, M. G. (1998) Nocturnal sleep and daytime somnolence in untreated patients with temporal lobe epilepsy: changes after treatment with controlled-release carbamazepine. *Epilepsia.* 38(6):676–701.

[11] Malow, B., Selwa, L. Ross, D., Aldrich, M. (1998). Lateralizing value of interictal spikes on overnight sleep-EEG studies in temporal lobe epilepsy, *Epilepsia.* 40(11):1592–1597.

[12] Bazil, C. W. & Walczak, T. S. (1998). Effects of sleep and sleep stage on epileptic and nonepileptic seizures, *Epilepsia* 38:69.

[13]   Bazil, C. W., Castro, L. H., Walczakt, T. S. (2000). Reduction of rapid eye movement sleep by diurnal and nocturnal seizures in temporal lobe epilepsy. *Archives of Neurology.* 57:363–368.

[14]   Roberts, R. (1998). Differential diagnosis of sleep disorders, non-epileptic attacks and epileptic seizures. *Current Opinion on Neurology.* 11:135-139.

[15]   Crespel, A., Coubes, P., Baldy-Molulinier, M. (2000). Sleep influence on seizures and epilepsy effects on sleep in partial frontal and temporal lobe epilepsies. *Clinical Neurophysiology.* 111(2):54-59.

[16]   Halász, P. (2013). How sleep activates epileptic networks? *Epilepsy Research and Treatment.* 425697:1-19.

[17]   Lothman, E. W. & Collins, R. C. (1981). Kainic acid induced limbic seizures: metabolic, behavioral, electroencephalographic and neuropathological correlates. *Brain Research.* 218:299–318.

[18]   Ng M. C. & Bianchi, M. T. (2014). Sleep misperception in patients with epilepsy. *Epilepsy and Behavior.* 36:9-11.

[19]   Berger, M., Gray, J. A., Roth, B. L. (2009). The expanded biology of serotonin. Annual Reviews on Medicine. 60:355-366.

[20]   Filip, M. & Bader, M. (2009). Overview on 5-HT receptors and their role in physiology and pathology on the central nervous system. *Pharmacological Reports.* 61:761-777.

[21]   Bardin, L. (2011). The complex role of serotonin and 5-HT receptors in chronic pain. *Behavioural Pharmacology.* 22:390-404.

[22]   Sakai, K. & Crochet, S. (2001). Differentiation of presumed serotonergic dorsal raphe neurons in relation to behavior and wake–sleep states. Neuroscience. 104:1141-1155.

[23]   Derry, C. P. & Duncan, S. (2013). Sleep and epilepsy. *Epilepsy & Behavior.* 26:394-404.

[24]   Cespuglio, R., Houdouin, F., Oulerich M.E., Mansari, M., Jouvet, M. (1990). Axonal and someto-dendritic modalities of serotonin release: their involvement in sleep preparation, triggering and maintenance. *Journal of Sleep Research.* 1:150-156.

[25]   Bouret, S. & Sara, S. J. (2005). Network reset: a simplified overarching theory of locus coeruleus noradrenaline function. Trends in *Neuroscience.* 28:574-582.

[26]   Hobson, J. A. & McCarley R. W. (1974). Selective firing by cat pontine stem neurons in desynchronized sleep. *Journal of Neurophysiology.* 37:1297-1299.

[27] Hobson, J. A., McCarley, R. W., Wyzinski, P. W. (1975). Sleep cycle oscillation reciprocal discharge by two brain neuronal groups. *Science.* 189:55-58.

[28] Vertes, R. P., Linley, S. B., Hoover, W. B. (2010). Pattern of distribution of serotoninergic fibers to the thalamus of the rat. *Brain Structure and Function.* 215:1-28.

[29] Koyama, Y. & Sakai, K. (2000). Modulation of presumed cholinergic mesopontine tegmental neurons by acetylcholine and monoamines applied iontophoretically in unanesthetized cats. *Neuroscience.* 96(4):723-733.

[30] Djordjevic, N., Milovanovic, D. D., Radovanovic, M., Radosavljevic, I., Obradovic, S., Jakovljevic, M., Milavanovic D., Milavanovic J.R., Jankovic S. (2016). CYP1A2 genotype affects Carbamazepine pharmacokinetics in children with epilepsy. *European Journal of Clinical Pharmacology.* Doi: 10.1007/s00228-015-2006-9.

[31] Ambrosio, A. F., Silva, A. P., Malva, J. O. (1999). Carbamazepine inhibits L-type Ca2$^+$ channels in culture rat hippocampal neurons stimulated with glutamate receptor agonists. *Neuropharmacology.* 38:1349–1350.

[32] Marksteiner, J. & Sperk G. (1988). Concomitant increase of somatostatin, neuropeptide y and glutamate decarylase in the frontal cortex of rats with decreased seizure threshold. *Neuroscience.* 26(2):379-385

[33] Faigle, J. W. & Feldman, K. F. (1982) *Antiepileptic drugs*, 2nd Edition (Woodbury, D.M.; Penry, J. K and pippenger, C.E.; Eds) Raven Press, New York.

[34] Hershkowitz, N., Dretchen, K., Raines, A. (1978). Carbamazepine suppression of postetanic potentiation at the neuromuscular junction. *Journal of Pharmacology and Experimental Therapeutics.* 207:810-816.

[35] Sperk, G. (1994). Kainic acid seizures in the rat. *Progress in Neurobiology.* 42:1-32.

[36] Shinozaki, H. & Jonishi, S. (1979). Actions of several antihelmintics and insecticides on rat cortical neurons. *Brain Research.* 24:368-371.

[37] Pollard, H., Héron, D., Moreau, J., Ben-Ari Y., Kherstchatisky, M. (1993). Alterations of the GluR-B AMP receptor subunit Flip/flop expression in Kainate-induced epilepsy and ischemia. *Neuroscience.* 57(3):545-554.

[38] Nadler, J. V. (1981). Kainic acid as tool for the study of temporal lobe epilepsy. *Life Sciences.* 29:165-167.

[39] Sperk, G. (1994). Kainic acid seizures in the rat. *Progress in Neurobiology.* 42:1-32.

[40] Zimmermann, M. (1983). Ethical guidelines for investigations of experimental pain in conscious animals. *Pain.* 16(2):109-110.

[41] Norma Oficial Mexicana. (1999). Especificaciones técnicas para la producción, cuidado y uso de los animales de laboratorio. NOM-062-ZOO-1999. [Official Mexican Normative. 1999. Technical specifications for production, care and use of laboratory animals. NOM-062-ZOO-1999].

[42] Alfaro-Rodríguez, A. & González-Piña, R. (2005). Ozone-induced paradoxical sleep decrease is related to diminished acetylcholine levels in the medial preoptic area in rats. *Chemico-Biological Interactions.* 151:151–158.

[43] Gibaldi, M. (1991). Compartamental and noncompartamental pharmacokinetics. In: Biopharmaceutics and clinical Pharmacokinetics. Lea and Febiger Editors. Philadelphia and London, fourth Edition, pp. 14-23.

[44] Akaike, K., Tanaka, H., Tojo, S., Fukumoto, S., Imamura, S., Takigawa, M. (2001). Kainic acid induced dorsal and ventral hippocampal seizures in rats. *Brain Research.* 900:65–71.

[45] Lothman, E. W. & Collins, R. C. (1981). Kainic acid induced limbic seizures: metabolic, behavioral, electroencephalographic and neuropathological correlates. *Brain Research.* 218:299-318.

[46] Ayala-Guerrero, F., Alfaro, A., Martínez, C., Campos-Sepúlveda, E., Vargas, L., Mexicano, G. (2002). Effect of Kainic Acid-Induced Seizures on Sleep Patterns. Proceedings of the Western Pharmacology. 45:178-180.

[47] Ferkany, J. W., Zaczek, R., Coyle, J. T. (1982). Kainic acid stimulates excitatory amino acid neurotransmitter release at presynaptic receptors. *Nature.* 298:757-759.

[48] Kölher, M., Burnashev, N., Sakmann, B., Seeburg, P.H. (1993). Determinants of ca2+ permeability in both TM1 and TM2 of high affinity kainate receptor channels: Diversity by RNA editing. *Neuron.* 10:491-500.

[49] Ben-Ari, Y., Trembalay, E., Richie, D., Ghilini, G., Naquet, R. (1981). Electrographic, cinical and pathological alterations following systemic administration of kainic acid, bicuculline of pentetrazole: Metabolic mapping using the deoxyglucose method with special reference to the pathology of epilepsy. *Neuroscience.* 6(7):1361-1391.

[50] Wade, J. V., Samson, F. E., Nelson, S. R., Pazdernik, T. L. (1987). Changes in Extracellular Amino Acids During Soman-and Kainic Acid-Induced Seizures. *Journal of Neurochemistry.* 49(2):645-650.

[51] Houser, C.R. (1991). Conductance rise induced by the calcium ionophore A23187 in unfertilized eggs of tilapia. *Experimental Physiology.* 76:619-22.

[52] Mendelson, W. B. & Monti, D. (1993). Do benzodiazepines induce sleep by a GABAergic mechanism? *Life Sciences.* 53:81-87.

[53] Poe, G. R., Nitz, D. A., McNaughton, B.L., Barnes, C.A. (2000). Experience-dependent phase-reversal of hippocampal neuron firing during REM sleep. *Brain Research.* 855:176-780.

[54] Schliebs R., Zivin, M., Steinbach, J., Rothe, T. (1989). Changes in cholinergic but not in GABAergic markers in amygdala, piriform cortex and nucleus basalis of the rat brain following systemic administration of kainic acid, *Journal of Neurochemistry.* 53:212–218.

[55] Fernández-Guardiola, A. (1992). Modelos experimentales de epilepsia. Gaceta Médica de México. 128:443-460. [Experimental models of epilepsy. (1992). *Medical Lancet of Mexico.* 128:443-460.]

[56] Degen, R., Rodin, E. A., *Epilepsy, Sleep and Sleep Deprivation.* 2nd Edition. Elsevier, Amsterdam, 1991.

[57] Taylor, C. P. (1996). Voltage-gated Na+ channel as targets for anticonvulsant, analgesic and neuroprotective drugs. *Current Pharmaceutical Design.* 2:375-388.

[58] Fern, R., Ramson, B. R., Stys, P. K., Waxman, S. G. (1993). Pharmacological protection of CNS whiter matter during anoxia: actions of phenytoin, carbamazepine and diazepam. *Journal of Pharmacology and Experimental Therapeutics.* 266:1549-1555.

[59] Rataud, J., Debarnot, F., Veronique, M., Pratt, J., Stutzmann, J. M. (1994). Comparative study of voltage-sensitive sodium channel blockers in focal ischemia and electric convolutions in rodents. *Neuroscience Letters.* 172:19-23.

[60] Minato, H., Kikuta, C., Fujitami, B., Masuda, Y. (1997). Protective effect of zonisamide an antiepileptic drug, against transient focal cerebral ischemia with middle cerebral artery occlusion reperfusion in rats. *Epilepsia.* 378:975-980.

[61] Waldmeier, P.C., Baumann, P. A., Wicki, P., Feldtrauer, J. J., Stierlin, C., Schmutz, M. (1995). Similar potency of carbamazepine, oxcarbamazepine, and lamotrigine in inhibiting the release of glutamate and other neurotransmitters. *Neurology.* 45(10):1907-1913.

BIOGRAPHICAL SKETCH

Alfonso Alfaro-Rodríguez

Affiliation: National Institute Of Rehabilitation, Mexico City, Mexico
Education:
-MD, Master Neurophysiological Sciences, of the Center of Neurobiology and Institute of Biomedical Research, Universidad Nacional Autónoma de México (UNAM).
-PhD (Neurosciences) Faculty of Sciences, Universidad Nacional Autónoma de México (UNAM).
Business Address: Av. Mexico-Xochimilco No. 289 Col. Arenal de Guadalupe, C.P. 14889 Mexico City, Mexico

Research and Professional Experience:

1987 to 1989 INCYTAS-DIF. Position: Research Assistant "C," Mexico City, Mexico
1990 to 1991 Researcher in the Department of Immunology and Malnutrition of the Unit of Research in Children's Health of the National Institute of Pediatrics of La Ssa. Position: Associate Investigator "C," Mexico City, Mexico.
1992 to 1996 Researcher in the Department of Biochemical Development of the Central Nervous System of the Child Health Research Unit of the National Institute of Pediatrics of La Ssa. Associate Investigator "C.," Mexico City, Mexico.
1996 to 2001 Researcher in the Department of Neurophysiology and Experimental Epilepsy of the National Institute of Neurology and Neurosurgery "Manuel Velasco Suarez," Mexico City, Mexico.
2001 to date Researcher in Medical Sciences "D," Responsible for the Division of Neurosciences, National Institute of Rehabilitation-SSA., Mexico City, Mexico.

Professional Appointments:

Professor of Thesis Seminar. Bachelor in Therapist in Human Communication. National Institute of Rehabilitation SSA., Mexico City, Mexico.

- Professor of Methods and Research Techniques in the Language and Hearing Masters at the National Institute of Rehabilitation SSA. Mexico City, Mexico
- Professor of Seminar of Thesis I and II in the Master of Speech and Hearing at the Institute of Human Communication. ., Mexico City, Mexico
- Professor of the subject Introduction to the Methodology of Research to Resident Physicians of the Specialty in Medicine in Human Communication, Audiology and Phoniatrics National Institute of Human Communication. Mexico City, Mexico
- Professor / Tutor of Masters and Doctorate, Postgraduate in Medical and Dental Health Sciences UNAM. ., Mexico City, Mexico
- Professor/Tutor of Masters, Postgraduate in Biological Sciences, Faculty of Sciences, UNAM. ., Mexico City, Mexico

Honors:

1. Diploma for having obtained the 2nd place at the XIII annual research meeting. National Institute of Neurology and Neurosurgery "MVS" SSA. May 1998.
2. Recognition for participation in the organizing committee of the second annual meeting of the National Rehabilitation Center, November 2002.
3. Recognition for participation in the organizing committee (scientific committee) of the third annual meeting: "Advances in the prevention, treatment and investigation of disability." National Rehabilitation Center SSA, November 2003.
4. Recognition for participation in the organizing committee (scientific committee) of the fourth annual meeting: "Current state and perspectives of research in disability." National Rehabilitation Center SSA, November 2004.
5. Acknowledgment of the Institute of Human Communication to the teaching work made in the licensee. May 2005.

6. Recognition as a Researcher in "D" Medical Sciences, -Secretary Health-National Coordination of Health Institutes, 2005.
7. Recognition of Scientific Productivity-Health Secretariat-National Coordination of Health Institutes, 2006.
8. Recognition of Scientific Productivity - Health Secretariat-National Coordination of Health Institutes, 2007.
9. Award "Acade. Dr. Francisco Fonseca García "To the 2nd Place. By work: Neurological effects of left common carotid ligation and hypoxia induced in neonatal rats-during the LXXV anniversary of the Mexican Academy of Surgery, November 25, 2008.
10. First place award with work: "Serotonin levels increase during motor deficit after sensoriomotor cortex injury in the rat." At the IX annual research meeting of the National Institute of Rehabilitation, held from November 18 to 20, 2009.
11. Prize to the second place with the work: "Serotonin levels increase during motor deficit after sensoriomotor cortex injury in the rat." At the II international meeting on rehabilitation, research of the National Institute of Rehabilitation held from November 18 to 20, 2011.
12. Recognition of scientific productivity - health secretariat-national coordination of Institutes De Salud, 2012.
13. Award "Acade. Dr. Francisco Fonseca García "To the 1st Place. By the work: Viability of parietal bone autograft preserved in adipose tissue. Preliminary report of an experimental study in rats. During the LXXX academic year of the Mexican Academy of Surgery, November 26, 2013.
14. Prize to the first place with the work: "Density profile of bone density assessed by computed tomography with determination by dual absorptiometry of DXA rays." At the VII international meeting on rehabilitation, research of the National Institute of Rehabilitation held from November 14 to 18, 2016.

Publications from the Last Three Years:

1. Soriano-Rosales RE, Perez-Guille BE, Arch-Tirado E, Alfaro-Rodriguez A, Villegas-Alvarez F, Gonzalez-Zamora JF, Jimenez-Bravo MA, Zaragoza-Huerta S, Gonzalez-Maciel A, Ramos-Morales A, Reynoso-Robles R, Mota-Rojas D (2014). Bioabsorbable implant as a tracheal wall substitute in young developing canines. ASAIO J. 2014 Jul-Aug; 60(4):466-72. ISSN: 1058-2916.

2. Solís-Chávez S A, Durand-Rivera A, Ibáñez-Contreras A, Reyes-Pantoja S A, Valderrama K, Heras-RomeroY, Tena-Betancourt E, Galván-Montaño A, Alfaro-Rodríguez A and Hernández-Godínez B (2014)Visual Evoked Potentials to Light Flashes in Captive Rhesus Monkeys: A Study Reflecting Cerebral Cortical Activity and Brain Maturation. Pak Vet J, 2014, 34(1): 41-45. ISSN: 0253-8318.

3. Fernández Cordova A, Gutierrez farfán I, Chamlati Aguirre E, Alfaro Rodríguez A, Durand Rivera A. (2014), Modificación de umbrales t en pacientes con implante coclear como una alternativa de programación en relación con el tiempo. Rev Invest Clin. 66(3), 247-251. . ISSN 0034-8376.

4. Alfonso Alfaro-Rodríguez, Javier Vargas-Sánchez, Cindy Bandala, Rebeca Uribe-Escamilla. (2014) Carbamazepine produces changes in the auditory pathway of Wistar rats. Rev Invest Clin. 66(4), pp345-350 ISSN 0034-8376.

5. Elizabeth Zambrano Sánchez; Yolanda del Río Carlos; Minerva Dehesa Moreno; Francisco Vázquez Urbano; Alfonso Alfaro Rodríguez (2014)"Terapia familiar sistémica en el tratamiento del trastorno por déficit de atención." Revista de Psicología Cientifica.Com ISSN: 2322-8644 Vol. 16 Año 2014. Publicado agosto 24 2014.

6. Guille García Sánchez, Alfonso Alfaro-Rodríguez, and Adrián Poblano (2014) "Evidence for Central Asian Origin of the p.Val27Ile Variant in the GJB2 Gene," International Journal of Medical Genetics, vol. 2014, Article ID 856313, 8 pages, 2014. doi:10.1155/ 2014/856313.

7. Elizabeth Zambrano-Sánchez, José A Martínez-Cortéz, Yolanda del Río-Carlos, Minerva Dehesa Moreno, Francisco Vázquez Urbano, Alfonso Alfaro Rodríguez (2015) Funciones ejecutivas en niños con TDAH de acuerdo con subtipo clínico y grupo control. Investigación en Discapacidad. Vol. 4, Núm. 1: pp 3-8. ISSN 2007-6452.

8. Avila-Luna A, Prieto-Leyva J, Gálvez-Rosas A, Alfaro-Rodriguez A, Gonzalez-Pina R, Bueno-Nava A. (2015) D1 Antagonists and D2 Agonists Have Opposite Effects on the Metabolism of Dopamine in the Rat Striatum. Neurochem Res. 40 (7):1431-7. ISSN: 0364-3190.

9. Angélica González-Maciel, Rosa María Romero-Velázquez, Rafael Reynoso-Robles, Rebeca Uribe-Escamilla, Javier Vargas- Sánchez, Paloma de la Garza Montaño, Alfonso Alfaro- Rodríguez (2015).

Prenatal protein malnutrition affects the density of GABAergic inter-neurons during hippocampus development in rats. Rev Invest Clin. 67(5): 296-303 ISSN: 2385-3956 *

10. Dela Garza-Montano P, Estrada-Villasenor E, Dominguez Rubio R, Martinez Lopez V, Avila-Luna A, Alfaro-Rodriguez A, Garciadiego-Cazares D, Carlos A, Hernandez-Perez AD, Bandala C (2015). Epidemiological aspects of musculoskeletal tumors (Osteosarcoma, Giant Cell Tumor and Chondrosarcoma): Experience of the National Institute of Rehabilitation, Mexico, City. Asian Pac J Cancer Prev. 2015;16(15):6451-6455. ISNN:1513-7368.

11. Bandala C, Terán-Melo J, Anaya-Ruiz M, Mejía-Barradas CM, Domínguez-Rubio R, De la Garza-Montaño P, Alfaro-Rodríguez A, Lara-Padilla E. (2015) Effect of botulinum neurotoxin type A (BoNTA) on the morphology and viability of 3T3 murine fibroblasts. Int J Clin Exp Pathol. 15;8(8):9458-9462 ISNN: 1936-2625.

12. Estrada-Villaseñor E, Uribe-Escamilla R, De la Garza-Montano P, Rubio R Dominguez, Martinez-Lopez V, Avila-Luna A, A Alfaro-Rodriguez, EK Ruvalcaba-Paredes, D Garciadiego-Cazares, C Bandala (2015) Association of Metastasis with Clinicopathological Data in Mexican Patients with Osteosarcoma, Giant Cell Tumor of Bone and Chondrosarcoma. Asian Pac J Cancer Prev.;16(17):7689-94. . ISNN:1513-7368.

13. Bandala Cindy, De la Garza-Montaño Paloma, Cortés-Algara Alfredo, Cruz- López Jaime, Domínguez-Rubio Rene, González-López Nelly Judith, Cárdenas- Rodríguez Noemi, Alfaro-Rodríguez A, Salcedo M, Floriano-Sanchez E, Lara-Padilla Eleazar (2015), Association of Histopathological Markers with Clinico- Pathological Factors in Mexican Women with Breast Cancer. Asian Pac J Cancer Prev.; 16 (18), 8397-8403 ISNN:1513-7368.

14. Lara-Padilla E, Miliar-Garcia A, Gomez-Lopez M, Romero-Morelos P, Bazan-Mendez C, Alfaro-Rodriguez A, Anaya-Ruiz M, Callender K, Carlos A, Bandala C. Neural Transdifferentiation: MAPTau Gene Expression in Breast Cancer Cells. Asian Pac J Cancer Prev. 2016;17(4):1967-71. ISNN:1513-7368.

15. Parada-Huerta E, Alvarez-Dominguez T, Uribe-Escamilla R, Rodriguez-Joya J, Ponce-Medrano JD, Padron-Lucio S, Alfaro-Rodriguez A, Bandala C.Metastasis Risk Reduction Related with Beta-Blocker Treatment in Mexican Women with Breast Cancer. Asian Pac J Cancer Prev. 2016;17(6):2953-7. ISNN:1513-7368.

16. Cortes-Altamirano JL, Olmos-Hernández A, Bonilla-Jaime H, Bandala C, González-Maciel A, Alfaro-Rodríguez A. Levetiracetam as an antiepileptic, neuroprotective, and hyperalgesic drug. Neurol India 2016;64:1266-75. ISNN : 0028-3886.

17. Alfredo Cortés-Algara, Noemí Cárdenas-Rodríguez, Eleazar Lara-Padilla, Esaú Floriano-Sánchez, Rebeca Martínez-Contreras, Maricruz Anaya-Ruiz, Rebeca Uribe-Escamilla, Alfonso Alfaro-Rodríguez, Ian Ilizaliturri-Flores, Martín Pérez-Santos, Cindy Bandala. Synaptic vesicle protein isoforms (SV2A, SV2B, SV2C): expression in breast cancer and their association with risk factors and metastasis in Mexican women. Int J Clin Exp Pathol 2017;10(2):1998-2004. ISSN:1936-2625.

In: Carbamazepine
Editor: Bernadette A. Woods

ISBN: 978-1-53611-954-1
© 2017 Nova Science Publishers, Inc.

Chapter 2

CARBAMAZEPINE IN SPORTS: A CALL FOR DISCUSSION

Borislav Radic[1],, Zoran Manojlovic[2] and Petra Radic[3]*
[1]Department of Neurology,
University Hospital Center Zagreb, Zagreb, Croatia
[2]Croatian Institute of Toxicology and Anti-Doping, Croatia
[3]School of Medicine, University of Zagreb,
Zagreb, Croatia

ABSTRACT

Doping in sport has been known since the Olympic Games in ancient Greece. Doping allows less capable athletes to achieve superior results. In non-Olympic sports doping is still poorly controlled. There have been reports on the use of carbamazepine in freediving. Carbamazepine produces the protective effect of hypoxia and prolongs latency for the development of convulsions and death. The World Anti-Doping Agency (WADA) and all organizations responsible for freediving started prohibiting the use of doping and implementing continuous monitoring, and thus enabled this beautiful activity to become an Olympic sport.

---

* E-mail: boris.radic105@gmail.com, Tel.: 01/2376-414, Mobile: 091/798-6045.

INTRODUCTION

Carbamazepine (Tegretol) is an antiepileptic from the carboxamide group with psychotropic and neurotropic effects. The antiepileptic activity of carbamazepine is based on increased glutamate release and the stabilization of neuronal membranes, whereas the decrease in dopaminergic and noradrenergic impulse conduction is responsible for its antimanic features. Carbamazepine also inhibits recurrent neuronal outbreaks, and the synaptic spread reduces excitatory pulses. It is assumed that the mechanism of action of carbamazepine is blocking sodium channels. It is used in the treatment of epilepsy as monotherapy as well as in combination with other antiepileptic drugs. Its psychotropic action provides better communication and resocialization for patients with epilepsy or bipolar disorder. Carbamazepine usually prevents the paroxysmal pain associated with idiopathic trigeminal neuralgia. In alcoholics with withdrawal syndrome it increases the threshold for seizure outbreaks of seizures and reduces withdrawal symptoms.

Doping is the use of prohibited substances and methods according to the current WADA Prohibed List. WADA and International Olympic Committee plays a crucial role in the fight against unfair means in sports, but it can be argued that IOC`s motto - "faster, higher, stronger" - may also be detrimental to sports, by turning recreation and entertainment into a merciless competition of individuals who are destroying their health in the desire for maximum profit and glory.

Even in ancient societies it was not unusual for some individuals to take certain substances that would enhance their performance. Most of them were warriors and athletes competing in the Olympic Games in ancient Greece [1]. However, this cannot be considered as doping, because such activities were neither prohibited nor uncommon.

The first instances of doping can be associated with horse races, because they were the first commercialized sport that attracted big money from betting. The use of performance-enhancing substances occurred due to the exhaustion of athletes while training for certain sports, and in a few instances even had a lethal outcome.

During the Second World War, a number of soldiers were given amphetamines (a type of stimulants which reduce fatigue and increase aggression), and German soldiers even received anabolic steroids. Later, many athletes started to use these substances to improve their results, removing the physical pain of the effort that accompanies sport. Many coaches give their athletes amphetamines to reduce the effect of fatigue and to increase aggressiveness in the game.

An increasing number of injuries, illnesses, and deaths led to the need to control substances that athletes were taking. The first doping controls at big sporting events were carried out during the 1968 Winter Olympic Games in Grenoble and the Summer Olympics in Mexico the same year. Doping was associated with athletes from the German Democratic Republic (GDR) and the People's Republic of China. Athletes from the GDR were given anabolic steroids on the national level in order to prove the superiority of the Aryan race. The use of substances was obvious since athletes from the GDR and the People's Republic of China achieved more records than all other countries. The use of doping in the GDR came to light when the Stasi (secret police of the GDR) records were made available, revealing that 10,000 athletes in the country had been receiving steroids [2, 3, 4]. The general trend among authorities and sporting organizations over the past several decades has been to strictly regulate the use of any substances that enhance any abilities of the athletes while playing their sports. Doping undermines health and therefore the ban on doping in sport is a most important task, aimong to preserve sports in their original intent to demonstrate individual performances based on sportsmen's and sportswomen's abilities and not on the type of doping. Anti-doping authorities state that using performance-enhancing drugs goes against the "spirit of sport".

For years now, the fight against doping in sport has been a strategic objective at global and national levels. The creation of policies and strategies for the fight against doping in sport involved countries, the International Olympic Committee, international sports federations, national sports associations, as well as various government and non-governmental bodies. Joint action resulted in the establishment of the World Anti-Doping Agency (WADA) in 1999, and the adoption of the World Anti-Doping Code in 2003. At the World Conference in Copenhagen in 2003, the World Anti-Doping Code was adopted as the basis for the fight against doping in sport throughout the world [5, 6].

Countries that adopted and signed the Copenhagen Declaration against Doping recognize and support the role of the WADA and its Code, and are committed to international and intergovernmental cooperation in harmonizing anti-doping policies and practices in sport.

DISCUSSION

Doping in sport remains a serious and complex issue, putting athletes' health at risk as well as jeopardizing the integrity and reputation of sport and its athletes who are clean. Specific substances and methods are banned for a reason. In the spirit of sport the use of doping is unacceptable, because doping allows less capable athletes to achieve superior results. Furthermore, doping harms athletes who play by the rules. Doping affects all levels of athletes. It could also affect future generations of athletes, who may be influenced by what top athletes do. The fight against doping requires a joint and comprehensive action to protect both the sport and the athletes, especially young ones. It is integral to the nature of sport itself that participants as well as spectators of all sports are confident that the competition is clean.

Although WADA is now taking great efforts to prevent doping in non-Olympic sports as well, uncontrolled doping intake is still possible. One of the affected sports is freediving. When questioning whether doping is present in competitive freediving, objective assessment is insufficient due to a lack of known facts. Since the beginning of doping control in freediving (Association Internationale pour le Developement de l' Apnee (AIDA, English: International Association for Developement of Apnea, 2000), Confederation Mondiale des Activites Subaquatiques (CMAS, English: World Underwater Fedaration, 2003)), only a few positive competitors have been discovered. Some indicators suggest that the "innocence" in freediving is only an illusion. This discussion aims to encourage appropriate institutions (national freediving federations, WADA) to take serious measures to prevent doping in freediving.

Prevention of doping should be taken seriously; otherwise, it quickly takes hold and leads to situations such as those witnessed in athletics and cycling. There are numerous examples from the Olympic Games in London of sports medals and cups being revoked. Unfortunately, many athletes today are taking doping in order to achieve the best possible results, as that brings financial gain and social status. The fight against doping requires money, and since freediving is not a commercial sport, there is the question of obtaining the necessary funds. Surely, passive observation will lead to the degradation of competitive freediving. There are several reasons for such a scenario. It is likely that some unscrupulous competitors will resort to doping to achieve superhuman results. In particular, this is possible in freediving, where doping control is inadequate or absent. As doping in extreme conditions and maximum apnea significantly increase the health risks that accompany doping, an increased number of diving incidents can be expected in freediving.

In the last few years we have seen extraordinary results - world records in freediving that other competitors could not even come close to. There was, for example, the world record at the AIDA in 2009 - 11 minutes and 35 seconds. AIDA and CMAS have occasional doping control (e.g., for beta blockers), but not for the antiepileptic drug carbamazepin. WADA does not have a list of prohibited substances acting on the extension of apnea in freediving. The doping control that is conducted is inappropriate and too general. As the duration of apnea is mostly determined by oxygen storage capability and the speed of oxygen consumption, it would seem that for freediving blood doping (EPO, blood transfusions) is the most effective type of doping. Blood doping significantly increases hemoglobin, thus increasing the storage of oxygen. Beta blockers reduce the heart rate dramatically.

The combination of these substances could extend apnea up to 30%. Strong doping is represented through the inhibition of neuronal excitation by antiepileptic drugs acting as sedatives with a muscle-relaxing effect. Carbamazepine has such an effect. Some experiments on mice have shown that adenosinergic agents such as adenosine, 2-chloroadenosine, N6-cyclohexyladenosine, dipyridamole, and carbamazepine produce the protective effect of hypoxia and prolong latency for the development of convulsions and death [7, 8, 9, 10]. CMAS does not control any substances or methods, whereas AIDA only occasionally tests for beta blockers, and samples are sent to a WADA certificated laboratories . Even if the testing detected a certain substance, the samples would still be approved as clean, considering that the drugs in question are not on the prohibited list. In other words, the most effective doping substances that prolong apnea are legal. The former president of AIDA, Bill Stromberg, said: "The point is not so much to stop cheating, as it is to protect athletes from substances that can be very dangerous in extreme apnea".

This debate could develop in two ways. At best, it could encourage responsible institutions to take appropriate measures in the fight for a healthy development of freediving. At worst, the information presented here might facilitate doping in freediving and entice even more competitors to enter a "contract with the devil".

Who is responsible? Responsibility lies in the hands of all athletes, national federations, international organizations, and WADA. They should use all the available knowledge, especially that obtained by scientific research, to make freediving an Olympic sport free of doping.

REFERENCES

[1] Kumar, Rajesh . Competing against doping. *Br. J. Sports Med.,* 2010; 44 (Suppl).

[2] "Sports Doping Statistics Reach Plateau in Germany". Deutsche Welle. 2003.

[3] Pain And Injury in Sport: Social And Ethical Analysis, Section III, Chapter 7, Page 111, by Sigmund Loland, Berit Skirstad, Ivan Waddington, Published by Routledge in 2006.

[4] Dynamo Liste (in German). 2002.

[5] Staff. Lausanne Declaration on Doping in Sport. 1999.

[6] Executive Committee at WADA official website, 2014.

[7] Hosseinzadeh H., Nassiri Asl M. Anticonvulsant, sedative and muscle relaxant effects of carbenoxolone in mice. *BMC Pharmacol.,* 2003; 3:3.

[8] Thorat S. N., Kulkarni S. K. The protective effect of adenosinergic agents, Ro 5-4864 and carbamazepine against hypoxic stress-induced neurotoxicity in mice. *Methods Find Exp. Clin. Pharmacol.,* 1990; 12(1):17-22.

[9] Thorat S. N. et al. Effect of MK-801 and Its Interaction With Adenosinergic Agents and Carbamazepine Against Hypoxic Stress-Induced Convulsions and Death in Mice. *Methods Find Exp. Clin. Pharmacol.,* 1990; 12 (9), 595-600.

[10] Thorat S. N., Kulkarni S. K. Benzodiazepine inverse agonist, DMCM- and peripheral agonist, Ro 5-4864-induced convulsions in mice: effect of adenosinergic agents. *Indian J. Exp. Biol.,* 1990; 28(12):1160-5.

In: Carbamazepine
Editor: Bernadette A. Woods

ISBN: 978-1-53611-954-1
© 2017 Nova Science Publishers, Inc.

Chapter 3

CARBAMAZEPINE IN THE ENVIRONMENT: SOURCES, FATE AND ADVERSE EFFECTS

A. Dordio[1,2,], V. Silva[1] and A. J. P. Carvalho[1,3]*

[1]Chemistry Department, School of Sciences and Technology,
University of Évora, Évora, Portugal
[2]MARE – Marine and Environmental Research Centre,
University of Évora, Évora, Portugal
[3]CQE – Évora Chemistry Centre,
University of Évora, Évora, Portugal

ABSTRACT

Carbamazepine is a largely prescribed drug worldwide but in the latest years has also become notoriously known as a ubiquitous contaminant of aquatic environments. Indeed, the frequent detection of carbamazepine in effluents of wastewater treatment plants is due to the general inefficiency of conventional wastewater treatment processes to remove this recalcitrant contaminant from incoming contaminated wastewaters. Several studies confirmed that carbamazepine is persistent to bio and photodegradation in the aquatic media and, due to its recalcitrant behaviour, it has been proposed as a possible anthropogenic marker in the aquatic environment. However, up until now only scarce information has been collected in regard to the potential ecological impacts of carbamazepine. It is, thus, very important to consolidate the

* Corresponding author: Tel: +351 - 266 745343; E-mail address: avbd@uevora.pt.

knowledge about its behaviour and fate in the environment and assess the risks it poses to aquatic ecosystems.

This work is a review of current reports on the presence of carbamazepine in the environment, complemented with a general overview of typical (usually low) efficiencies with which conventional wastewater treatment plants are capable of removing carbamazepine from domestic wastewaters. Furthermore, processes and influencing factors that determine the fate of carbamazepine in wastewater treatment plants and in the environment are presented and discussed. Finally, various technologies that have been under study and development over recent years in response to the general inefficiency of conventional wastewater treatment processes in treating carbamazapine and other emerging pollutants are outline and discussed briefly. Hopefully, prospects for significant improvements in carbamazepine removal efficiencies and potential means to achieve that goal in the future are pointed out in this work.

1. INTRODUCTION

As a side effect of the widespread use of pharmaceuticals in modern society, their residues are being detected with ever increasing regularity in analyses of environmental samples worldwide (Fent et al., 2006; Aga, 2008; Caliman and Gavrilescu, 2009; Fatta-Kassinos et al., 2011; Lapworth et al., 2012; Luo et al., 2014; Li, 2014; Gavrilescu et al., 2015; Sui et al., 2015; Petrie et al., 2016; Mohapatra et al., 2016; Ebele et al., 2017; Archer et al., 2017). In fact, a growing number of environmental studies conducted at diverse locations of the planet have been reporting the detection of several pharmaceuticals, their metabolites and transformation products, albeit usually at very low concentrations (in the $\mu g\ L^{-1}$ to $ng\ L^{-1}$ levels), in sewage sludges, soils, raw and treated wastewaters, receiving water bodies, groundwater and even in drinking water (Fent et al., 2006; Zhang et al., 2008; Bolong et al., 2009; Calisto and Esteves, 2009; Fatta-Kassinos et al., 2011; Lapworth et al., 2012; Verlicchi et al., 2012; Rivera-Utrilla et al., 2013; Li, 2014; Evgenidou et al., 2015; Sui et al., 2015; Verlicchi and Zambello, 2015; Sun et al., 2015; García-Santiago et al., 2016; Noguera-Oviedo and Aga, 2016; Ebele et al., 2017). The adverse effects of these pharmaceutical residues to the environment and their impact on living organisms is largely yet to be assessed. However, considering the targets and functions of these substances, which are designed to interfere with biological and biochemical processes, there seems to be a potential for perturbation of normal natural processes. In fact, there is some evidence that a continuous exposure to even some low levels of certain pharmaceuticals may in the long term have both acute and chronic effects on various organisms, as well as potential indirect effects on ecosystems (Boxall, 2004; Fent et al., 2006; Farré et al., 2008; Bolong et al., 2009; Calisto and Esteves, 2009; Pal et al., 2010; Santos et al., 2010; Escher et al., 2011; Du and Liu, 2012; Kumar et al., 2012a; Zenker et al., 2014; Arnold et al., 2014; Barra Caracciolo et al., 2015; Godoy et al., 2015; Ebele et al., 2017).

Over the last years, a large and sometimes unexpected variety of sources and routes has been identified through which pharmaceuticals may enter in and be distributed through various environmental compartments (Halling-Sørensen et al., 1998; Heberer, 2002; Farré et al., 2008; Lapworth et al., 2012; Lees et al., 2016; Ebele et al., 2017). Among these, wastewater point sources are widely considered as the primary route of entry for pharmaceuticals, their metabolites or transformation products in the environment (Fent et al., 2006; Aga, 2008; Bolong et al., 2009; Verlicchi et al., 2012; Luo et al., 2014; Evgenidou et al., 2015; Noguera-Oviedo and Aga, 2016). They are introduced in the wastewater treatment plants (WWTPs) in result of excretion of ingested/administered medication either in non-metabolized form (i.e., the portion that is not absorbed by the body) or in the form of various metabolites. In addition to this main source, there is frequently an also significant contribution resulting from improper disposal of expired medications. Meanwhile, the fate of these substances in WWTPs corresponds in many cases to removal or transformation of only a minor portion of these pollutants. The problem is that conventional WWTPs are generally designed to treat bulk pollutants and the wastewater treatment processes used in such plants for such purpose are not the most efficient to also remove micropollutants (such as pharmaceutical residues) (Fatta-Kassinos et al., 2011; Verlicchi et al., 2012; Luo et al., 2014; Gavrilescu et al., 2015; Evgenidou et al., 2015). In fact, conventional WWTPs are frequently very inefficient towards micropollutants' cleanup, which leads to a significant fraction of the pharmaceuticals and their metabolites in the WWTP's influent being discharged with the final effluent into the receiving water bodies. Furthermore, as treated wastewaters are increasingly being reused for certain applications such as irrigation, as well as sewage sludge/biosolids being applied to land used in agriculture and forestry, a serious issue may be developing in regard to the contamination of soils with pharmaceuticals (Chenxi et al., 2008; Nieto et al., 2010; Walters et al., 2010; Du and Liu, 2012; Li, 2014; Durán-Álvarez et al., 2015; García-Santiago et al., 2016; Paz et al., 2016; Mohapatra et al., 2016; Lees et al., 2016). Ensuing the introduction of pharmaceuticals in the soil, contamination of surface water by run-off or of groundwater by leaching may aggravate and disseminate the problem. Moreover, as some of these substances also have the potential of being taken up by plants that are being cultivated or naturally grow on such contaminated soils, there is a risk that crops can also become contaminated and, subsequently, ingested by herbivores and be passed along the food chain (Carter et al., 2014; Wu et al., 2015; Paz et al., 2016; Ebele et al., 2017; Bartrons and Peñuelas, 2017). Hence, there is some potential for these practices to become a widespread environmental and public health problem, instead of the environmental benefits they were aiming to provide.

Carbamazepine is a widely prescribed drug and is also a well-known ubiquitous contaminant of municipal WWTPs effluents, receiving water bodies, soils, sediments and plants (Miao and Metcalfe, 2003; Clara et al., 2004b; Miao et al., 2005; Zhang et al., 2008; Leclercq et al., 2009; Luo et al., 2014; Bahlmann et al., 2014; Li, 2014; Durán-Álvarez et al., 2015; Petrie et al., 2016; Paz et al., 2016; Papageorgiou et al., 2016; Meyer et al., 2016; Archer et al., 2017).

After oral administration, 72% of the ingested dose of carbamazepine is absorbed and excreted in the urine while 28% is eliminated in the faeces (Miao and Metcalfe, 2003; Miao et al., 2005; Zhang et al., 2008; Petrovic et al., 2009; Bahlmann et al., 2014; Evgenidou et al., 2015). Once absorbed, carbamazepine is extensively metabolized by the human liver, with more than thirty metabolites having been already identified in human urine (Miao and Metcalfe, 2003; Miao et al., 2005; Leclercq et al., 2009; Bahlmann et al., 2014; Evgenidou et al., 2015). Data from pharmacokinetic studies allow to assess that only 1–2% of the total absorbed amount of carbamazepine is subsequently excreted in a non-metabolized form (Miao and Metcalfe, 2003; Miao et al., 2005; Petrovic et al., 2009; Bahlmann et al., 2014). However, the glucuronide conjugates of carbamazepine can presumably be cleaved in the sewage, which restores the conjugated compound into its original free form and, thereby, may increase carbamazepine concentrations in the final WWTP effluent (Ternes, 1998; Vieno et al., 2006; Vieno et al., 2007; Zhang et al., 2008; Petrovic et al., 2009; Leclercq et al., 2009; Zorita et al., 2009; Bahlmann et al., 2014; Evgenidou et al., 2015). In addition, carbamazepine excreted with faeces is probably partly enclosed in faeces particles and released during biological treatment, thereby contributing to augment its final concentration in the WWTP effluent (Luo et al., 2014; Blair et al., 2015).

Carbamazepine is very persistent and little to no degradation during conventional wastewater treatment with activated sludge takes place (Clara et al., 2004b; Vieno et al., 2007; Zhang et al., 2008; Celiz et al., 2009; Luo et al.,

2014; Bahlmann et al., 2014). Due to its recalcitrant nature and its high ubiquity in the environment, carbamazepine has already been proposed as an anthropogenic marker for the contamination of the aquatic environment (Clara et al., 2004b; Jekel et al., 2015; König et al., 2016). In fact, this pharmaceutical is among the most frequently detected in WWTPs effluents, at relatively high concentrations which may reach as high as 1 mg L^{-1} (Metcalfe et al., 2003; Clara et al., 2004b; Zhang et al., 2008; Verlicchi et al., 2012; Bahlmann et al., 2014; Gracia-Lor et al., 2014; Paz et al., 2016).

Up until now only scarce information has been gathered on potential ecotoxicological impacts attributable to carbamazepine. However, chronic effects have already been identified resulting from exposure to carbamazepine at environmentally relevant concentrations which include altered behavior, reduced immune response, and changes in growth and fecundity (Quinn et al., 2008; Martin-Diaz et al., 2009; van den Brandhof and Montforts, 2010; Contardo-Jara et al., 2011; Li et al., 2011; Gust et al., 2013; Brandão et al., 2013; Lamichhane et al., 2013; Jarvis et al., 2014; Mohapatra et al., 2014). In addition carbamazepine-related teratogenic effects have been observed clinically (Ternes et al., 2004b) and several researchers have speculated that the teratogenic effects associated with carbamazepine exposure are due to its metabolites rather than the parent compound (Miao et al., 2005; Leclercq et al., 2009; Celiz et al., 2009; Bahlmann et al., 2014). Furthermore, ecotoxicity of carbamazepine metabolites is even more poorly characterized, but the important metabolite CBZ-DiOH has been shown to possess similar anti-epileptic properties to carbamazepine, and it may cause neurotoxic effects (Miao et al., 2005; Celiz et al., 2009). In some cases, clinical toxicities parallel the also important metabolite CBZ-EP concentration (Miao et al., 2005).

Considering the recalcitrant character and potential ecotoxicity of carbamazepine and its metabolites, it is, thus, very important to consolidate the knowledge about the behaviour and fate of these compounds in the environment and to assess the risks they may pose to aquatic ecosystems.

In this work we aim to review some of the most current data available relating to the presence and fate of carbamazepine in the environment as well as to characterize the efficiencies of conventional WWTPs in removing carbamazepine from domestic wastewaters. Finally, a brief overview will be presented of the research work that has been carried out over the latest years to attempt significant improvements of carbamazepine removal efficiencies through the optimization of conventional wastewater treatment processes or the development of alternative/complementary wastewater treatment processes.

2. OCCURRENCE OF CARBAMAZEPINE
IN THE AQUATIC ENVIRONMENT

Carbamazepine is a notorious case among pharmaceutical pollutants as it is repeatedly detected among the contaminants of aquatic environmental samples in monitoring studies. This circumstance is due to its long history of clinical usage and to its outstandingly recalcitrant behavior (Clara et al., 2004b; Zhang et al., 2008; Luo et al., 2014; Bahlmann et al., 2014; Li, 2014; Gavrilescu et al., 2015). In fact, due to its persistence in the environment carbamazepine has been proposed as a suitable marker for anthropogenic influences on the aquatic environment (Clara et al., 2004b; Jekel et al., 2015; König et al., 2016).

Table 1 presents a summary of recent data available in the literature on the occurrence of carbamazepine in various types of water resources, in WWTPs effluents and sludge samples.

A brief overview of Table 1 reveals that, typically, carbamazepine is detected in WWTPs effluents, surface and ground waters, and occasionally in drinking water at concentration levels in the range of ng L^{-1} to μg L^{-1}. The concentration levels at which carbamazepine is detected in each type of medium is typically descending from WWTP effluents, to surface waters, to groundwater and finally in drinking water, which can be understood as result of dilution and of some elimination/transformation processes (such as retention in soil or photodegradation) as carbamazepine transfers from one aquatic medium to the other.

In addition to aquatic media, carbamazepine has also been detected in sewage sludge, typically at concentration levels of ng/g_{dw}.

Due to increasing reuse of treated wastewater for irrigation as well as the application of sewage sludge (biosolids) in soils as fertilizer or compost, carbamazepine has also been detected in plants grown at contaminated soils (Wu et al., 2010; Herklotz et al., 2010; Tanoue et al., 2012; Sabourin et al., 2012; Wu et al., 2012; Calderón-Preciado et al., 2013; Carter et al., 2014; Wu et al., 2014; Paz et al., 2016). Furthermore, runoff and leaching waters at such contaminated soils also contribute to the contamination of surface and groundwater with carbamazepine (Sabourin et al., 2009; Katz et al., 2009; Gibson et al., 2010; Gottschall et al., 2012; Bondarenko et al., 2012; Wu et al., 2015).

Table 1. Occurrence of carbamazepine residues in WWTP effluents and sludges and in the aquatic environment (values inside brackets are average values)

Surface water (ng/L)	Groundwater (ng/L)	Drinking water (ng/L)	WWTPs effluent (ng/L)	Sewage sludge (biosolids) (ng/g_{dw})	Reference
(250)	-	-	(2100)	-	(Ternes, 1998)
(7)	-	-	(426.2)	-	(Miao and Metcalfe, 2003)
60–1500	-	258	-	-	(Stackelberg et al., 2004)
< (8)	< (6)	< (6)	(420)	-	(Lin et al., 2005)
-	-	-	-	(69.6)	(Miao et al., 2005)
-	-	-	(410)	-	(Petrovic et al., 2005)
(24.56)	14–43	-	160–290	-	(Rabiet et al., 2006)
-	-	-	< 70–300 (160)	-	(Gómez et al., 2007)
4.5–61 (25)	-	-	73–729 (226)	-	(Kim et al., 2007)
-	-	-	13–110 (52)	-	(Martínez Bueno et al., 2007)
-	-	-	-	ND–215	(Nieto et al., 2007)
-	-	-	290-2440 (720)	-	(Vieno et al., 2007)
-	-	-	-	(34.5)	(Chenxi et al., 2008)
BDL–36	-	-	BDL–195	-	(Choi et al., 2008)
102–1194	-	-	-	-	(Reinstorf et al., 2008)
0.5–647	-	-	152–4596	-	(Kasprzyk-Hordern et al., 2009)
-	-	-	150-2300 (674)	-	(Miège et al., 2009)
-	-	-	-	(79.8)	(Radjenovic et al., 2009)
-	-	-	BDL–1.55	-	(Santos et al., 2009)
-	-	-	69–2377	-	(Huerta-Fontela et al., 2010)
-	-	-	-	12–42	(Nieto et al., 2010)
-	-	-	40–74 (55)	-	(Behera et al., 2011)
749 max	-	601 max	-	-	(Kleywegt et al., 2011)

Table 1. (Continued)

Surface water (ng/L)	Groundwater (ng/L)	Drinking water (ng/L)	WWTPs effluent (ng/L)	Sewage sludge (biosolids) (ng/g$_{dw}$)	Reference
82 max	-	-	-	-	(Spongberg et al., 2011)
ND–31.6	-	-	-	-	(Vulliet et al., 2011)
ND-9.6	-	ND-4.7	-	-	(Wang et al., 2011)
-	23.9-62.4	-	10-107	-	(Cabeza et al., 2012)
-	-	-	(713)	(164)	(Lajeunesse et al., 2012)
BQL-90	BQL-35	-	269 max	-	(Wolf et al., 2012)
-	-	-	-	60.6–371	(Yu and Wu, 2012)
	60-61		123-369		(Calderón-Preciado et al., 2013)
-	BQL-136	-	-	-	(López-Serna et al., 2013)
2–26 (9)	-	-	430–2760 (1010)	-	(Gracia-Lor et al., 2014)
-	(3.4)	-	-	-	(Petrovic et al., 2014)
-	BDL–41	-	-	-	(Radovic et al., 2014)
-	BQL–72	-	-	-	(Schaider et al., 2014)
-	BQL–9.3	-	-	-	(Tran et al., 2014)
(17.2)	-	-	(193)	-	(Durán-Álvarez et al., 2015)
-	-	-	-	18–113	(Gago-Ferrero et al., 2015)
-	0.4–37.9	-	-	-	(Lin et al., 2015)
-	-	-	91.3–731	28.6–191	(Subedi and Kannan, 2015)
(75.8)	-	-	(316)	(121)	(Petrie et al., 2016)
-	-	-	(580)	(22)	(Subedi et al., 2017)

BDL: below the detection limit; BQL: below the quantification limit; ND: not detected; max: maximum value of several determinations.

There is also some evidence of carbamazepine contamination of the biota of receiving water bodies/aquatic ecosystems (Ferrari et al., 2003; Oetken et al., 2005; Celiz et al., 2009; Huerta et al., 2012; Jarvis et al., 2014; Almeida et al., 2014; Valdés et al., 2014).

From the analysis of the data in Table 1 it also stands out that reported concentration levels of carbamazepine vary significantly, even in a similar aquatic medium. This variability results from the fact that concentrations are typically low and strongly affected by many factors which vary both in terms spatial location and in time. This includes world distribution and seasonal variations of production/sales/consumption levels, thus affecting WWTPs inputs, as well as some aspects that relate with WWTP design and operation that affect the characteristics of the final WWTP effluent (water consumption per person and per day, environmental conditions, WWTP size, plant configuration especially the type of bioreactor, hydraulic retention time, solids retention time).

The diversity of locations at which studies referred in Table 1 have been conducted show that contamination with carbamazepine is widespread throughout several countries in different continents and, therefore, it is a worldwide issue.

3. SOURCES, FATE AND EFFECTS OF CARBAMAZEPINE IN ENVIRONMENT

Research on the presence of pharmaceuticals in the environment has established, so far, a large and sometimes unexpected variety of routes through which these contaminants cross and are distributed to various environmental compartments. Figure 1 presents a scheme of possible pathways for entry and fate of carbamazepine, their metabolites and other transformation/degradation products in the environment.

Since anti-epileptic drug carbamazepine is used in the treatment of epilepsy and anxiety, hospital and domestic wastewaters are regarded as the primary route of entry of carbamazepine and its metabolites and transformation products in the environment (Clara et al., 2004b; Miao et al., 2005; Zhang et al., 2008; Leclercq et al., 2009; Santos et al., 2013; Yuan et al., 2013; Bahlmann et al., 2014; Subedi and Kannan, 2015; Verlicchi et al., 2015; de Almeida et al., 2015; Azuma et al., 2016). Carbamazepine enters the sewage system when the ingested drug is excreted, either in a non-metabolized form or as one of its metabolites. In addition, another significant source of carbamazepine in the sewage system results from the inadequate disposal of expired packages.

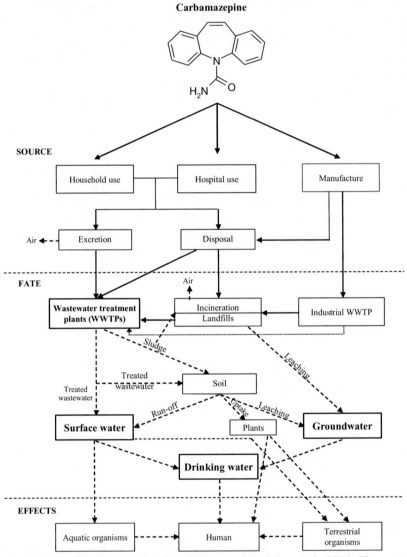

Sources: Halling-Sørensen et al., 1998; Heberer, 2002; Miao et al., 2005; Zhang et al., 2008; Farré et al., 2008; Lapworth et al., 2012; Bahlmann et al., 2014.

Figure 1. Sources, pathways, fate and impacts of carbamazepine.

In regard to the ingested compound, about 72% of the administered dose is absorbed by the body and is subsequently excreted in the urine in various forms. The remainder 28% is not absorbed and is eliminated in the faeces (Miao and Metcalfe, 2003; Miao et al., 2005; Zhang et al., 2008; Petrovic et al., 2009; Bahlmann et al., 2014; Evgenidou et al., 2015). Once inside the organism/body, carbamazepine is subjected to extensive hepatic metabolization, with more than 30 metabolites having been already identified, which, according to available studies, are excreted mainly via urine (Figure 2) (Miao et al., 2005; Zhang et al., 2008; Leclercq et al., 2009; Bahlmann et al., 2014; Evgenidou et al., 2015). According to relevant reports (Miao and Metcalfe, 2003; Miao et al., 2005; Zhang et al., 2008; Petrovic et al., 2009; Bahlmann et al., 2014), from the absorbed dose of carbamazepine that is excreted via urine, only about 1% consists of the parent compound (Miao et al., 2005; Zhang et al., 2008; Bahlmann et al., 2014). Therefore, nearly all the non-metabolized carbamazepine is excreted via faeces. Among all the carbamazepine metabolites that are present in urine, the most relevant metabolites are 10,11-dihydro-10,11-dihydroxycarbamazepine (CBZ-DiOH), which is not therapeutically active, and to a lesser extent 10,11-dihydro-10,11-epoxycarbamazepine (CBZ-EP). The latter possesses similar anti-epileptic properties to carbamazepine and may cause neurotoxic effects (Miao et al., 2005). Albeit being chemically stable under physiological conditions, CBZ-EP may be converted to CBZ-DiOH by the epoxide hydrolase enzyme. Other also relevant metabolites include 2-hydroxycarbamazepine (CBZ-2OH), 3-hydroxycarbamazepine (CBZ-3OH) and 10,11-dihydro-10-hydroxycarbamazepine (CBZ-10OH). Carbamazepine and some of its metabolites have been found to be partially excreted as glucuronide conjugates (either N-glucuronides or O-glucuronides, depending on the parent compound), although some of these conjugates may potentially be cleaved in the sewage and restored back to their parent free form (Zhang et al., 2008; Bahlmann et al., 2014).

The fate of carbamazepine and some of its metabolites in WWTPs in many cases corresponds to only some minor removal or transformation because conventional WWTPs are mostly inefficient to remove carbamazepine and its metabolites (Miao and Metcalfe, 2003; Metcalfe et al., 2003; Spongberg and Witter, 2008; Leclercq et al., 2009; Lajeunesse et al., 2012; Lapworth et al., 2012; Bahlmann et al., 2014; Hapeshi et al., 2015; Petrie et al., 2016; Subedi et al., 2017). Therefore, these compounds are usually still present in effluents from WWTPs, which represent the most important point source of contamination of surface waters.

Other possible sources of aquatic contamination with carbamazepine are the wastewaters of the pharmaceutical industry, leakages in wastewater treatment systems and landfill leachates (Sim et al., 2011; Bondarenko et al., 2012; Masoner et al., 2014; Clarke et al., 2015; Ramakrishnan et al., 2015; Lu et al., 2016; Masoner et al., 2016; Sui et al., 2017).

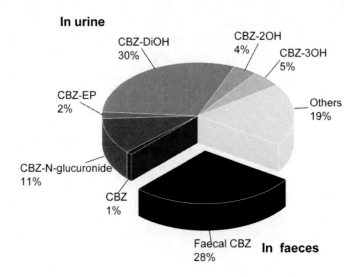

Figure 2. Carbamazepine (CBZ) and some of its metabolites and their percentual proportions in excreted amounts (adapted from Zhang et al. (2008) and Bahlmann et al. (2014)).

Additionally, some studies report the occurrence of contamination of soils (especially agricultural ones) with carbamazepine which is mainly caused by irrigation with treated wastewaters and from the use of sewage sludge (biosolids) as fertilizer or compost (Li et al., 2013; Li, 2014; Aznar et al., 2014; Al Rajab et al., 2015; Petrie et al., 2016; Paz et al., 2016; Mohapatra et al., 2016). The presence of pharmaceuticals in soil may extend contamination to surface waters by run-off or of groundwaters by leaching. In fact, carbamazepine has been frequently detected in leachates or runoff from land that had been irrigated with treated wastewater (Sabourin et al., 2009; Katz et al., 2009; Gibson et al., 2010; Gottschall et al., 2012; Bondarenko et al., 2012; Wu et al., 2015), implying a high mobility of carbamazepine in soil. Carbamazepine is highly persistent in soils and has long half-life times (Löffler et al., 2005; Walters et al., 2010; Li et al., 2013).

Furthermore, some studies report that carbamazepine has the potential to be taken up by plants which spontaneously grow or are cultivated over contaminated soils (Wu et al., 2010; Herklotz et al., 2010; Tanoue et al., 2012; Sabourin et al., 2012; Wu et al., 2012; Calderón-Preciado et al., 2013; Carter et al., 2014; Carvalho et al., 2014; Wu et al., 2014; Paz et al., 2016; Bartrons and Peñuelas, 2017). There is, therefore, a non-negligible possibility that crops can also become contaminated, thus posing a public health risk. In fact, the chance that vegetation uptakes and accumulates pharmaceuticals like carbamazepine suggests a risk that it will take part of the diet of herbivores and, subsequently, be passed along the food chain.

Finally, in regard to the risks posed to human health, carbamazepine has also been detected in tap water, which may be due to its frequent presence in water bodies that may serve as supplies of drinking water and, thus, also showing that drinking water treatment in some cases may not be entirely efficient in removing this pollutant from water (Stackelberg et al., 2004; Rivera-Utrilla et al., 2013; Sun et al., 2015; Simazaki et al., 2015). This opens up the possibility that there might be in some cases a direct exposure of human populations to carbamazepine.

3.1. Biotic and Abiotic Processes Involved in the Fate of Carbamazepine

Before and after carbamazepine reaches environmental compartments it is subjected to both biotic and abiotic processes responsible for its transport, transfer and transformation/degradation. The most important processes responsible for the fate of carbamazepine in water and wastewater treatment plants and in the environmental compartments are presented in Figure 3.

The main processes involved in organic pollutant transformation/degradation, retention or transfer between compartments may include sorption, hydrolysis, biological transformation/degradation, redox reactions, photodegradation, volatilization and precipitation/solubilization (Fent et al., 2006; Aga, 2008; Farré et al., 2008; Kasprzyk-Hordern, 2010; Luo et al., 2014; Li, 2014; Sui et al., 2015; Ebele et al., 2017; Archer et al., 2017). These processes occur continuously and concomitantly. Some of them can be competitive (e.g., photolysis and adsorption to soil) or even antagonistic (e.g., leaching and degradation). Overall, they influence the presence and mobility of pollutants. The response of carbamazepine to any of these pathways for partitioning, degradation or transformation in environmental compartments and in water/wastewater treatment plants may contribute to reduce its concentration in the environment and thereby reduce its potential to impact human health and aquatic life.

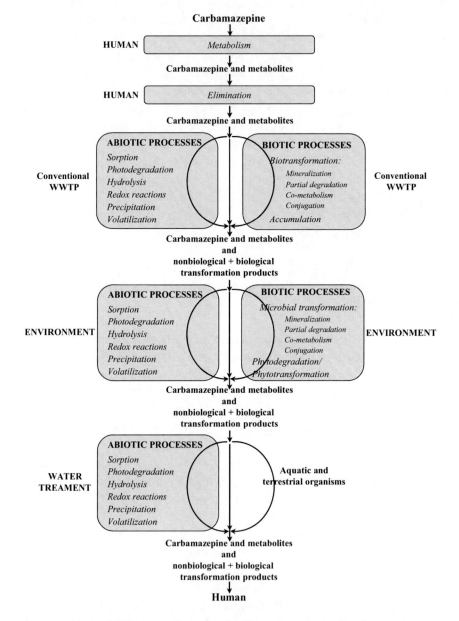

Figure 3. Abiotic and biotic processes involved in carbamazepine fate in aquatic environments (adapted from Barbara Kasprzyk-Hordern (2010)).

Given some of the common characteristics of the physical and chemical behavior of many pharmaceuticals, the abiotic processes that are most likely to transform them and to more permanently remove them from the aquatic environment include hydrolysis and photodegradation (Petrovic and Barceló, 2007; Aga, 2008; Kümmerer, 2008; Li, 2014). However, considering the passage of pharmaceuticals through the digestive tract and their relatively long-residence time in aqueous environments within WWTPs, hydrolysis reactions will likely play a less important role in the aquatic fate of many pharmaceuticals that reach the environment (Arnold and McNeill, 2007). On the other hand, direct photodegradation by sunlight may be an important elimination process for pharmaceuticals with absorbances in the 290-800 nm region of the radiation spectrum (Velagaleti, 1997; Andreozzi et al., 2003). In any case, the extent to which any of the several abiotic and biotic processes may potentially influence the short-term behavior and long-term fate of a pharmaceutical in the environment and water treatment systems is controlled by many factors related both with the pharmaceutical properties and with the environmental conditions.

Some of the most important properties of carbamazepine and of some of its metabolites, with relevance for their fate in the environment and in wastewater/water treatment systems, are presented in Table 2.

Carbamazepine metabolites are relatively poorly characterized in comparison with their parent compound carbamazepine and information on their properties is scarce or mostly unavailable.

From the available data, as presented in Table 2, it is clear that carbamazepine's properties make it a quite persistent pollutant and hard to degrade by natural processes in both compartments, water and soil, as can be assessed by its half-life for abiotic degradation (hydrolysis, photolysis) and biodegradation in the range of months (in water) to years (in soil). In particular, concerning biodegradation, its value of the biodegradation rate constant k_{biol} is too low according to the classification scheme for pollutants biodegradability. Contaminants can be classified according to their k_{biol} into very highly ($k_{biol} > 5$ L g_{ss}^{-1} d^{-1}), highly ($1 < k_{biol} < 5$ L g_{ss}^{-1} d^{-1}), moderately ($0.5 < k_{biol} < 1$ L g_{ss}^{-1} d^{-1}) or hardly biodegradable ($k_{biol} < 0.5$ L g_{ss}^{-1} d^{-1}) (Joss et al., 2006; Suarez et al., 2010; Kruglova et al., 2014) and carbamazepine clearly is part of the latter group. Therefore, low removal efficiencies are to be expected during biological treatment in WWTPs.

Table 2. Relevant physical and chemical properties of carbamazepine and of some of its metabolites

Compound		CBZ	CBZ-EP	CBZ-2 OH	CBZ-10 OH	CBZ-DiOH
Structure						
Molecular weight (g mol^{-1})		236.3	252.3	252.3	254.3	270.3
Henry's law const. 25°C (atm m^{3}mol^{-1})		1.08×10^{-10} [a,b]				
Water solubility (mg L^{-1})		17.7(estimated) [c] 112 [d]	1340 [e]	120 [e]		290 [e]
pKa		13.9 [f], 14 [g]	15.96 [e]	9.3 [h] 9.15 [e]	14 [h]	8.24 [e]
log K_{ow}		2.25 [i], 2.67 [i] 2.45 [a], 2.77 [j]	1.26 [i], 1.97 [h,j]	2.25 [i], 2.66 [h]	0.93 [i], 1.73 [h]	0.13 [i], 0.81 [j]
Partition coefficient log K_d	Sludge	1.633 [k], < 1.3 PS [l,m] (0.08-0.09 SS) [l,m]	-	-	-	-
	Soil	1.114 [k], 1.57 [n,o] (2.00 − 3.42) [g] (2.24 − 2.27) [p]	-	-	-	-
Half-Life (days)	Soil	462-533 [q] 328 [r], > 120 [s]	-	-	-	-
	Water	38 [t], 63 [u]				
Biodegradation rate constant k_{biol} (L g$_{SS}$$^{-1}$ d^{-1})		< 0.06 [v], 0.2 [w]	-	-	-	-

PS: primary sludge; SS: secondary sludge.

Sources: a: (SRC, 2009); b: (Zhang et al., 2008); c: (Meylan et al., 1996); d: (Ferrari et al., 2003); e:(DrugBank, 2017); f: (Jones et al., 2002); g: (Scheytt et al., 2005); h: (Lee et al., 2013); i:(Miao et al., 2005); j: (Paz et al., 2016); k:(Barron et al., 2009); l:(Ternes et al., 2004a); m: (Maurer et al., 2007); n: (Beausse, 2004); o: (Drillia et al., 2005); p: (Scheytt et al., 2004); q: (Walters et al., 2010); r: (Löffler et al., 2005); s: (Li et al., 2013); t: (Andreozzi et al., 2002); u: (Tixier et al., 2003); v:(Suarez et al., 2010); w:(Kruglova et al., 2014).

Photodegradation is also quite slow for carbamazepine, which seems to be relatively persistent towards direct photolysis. Indirect photolysis in most cases increased degradation rates. Humic material has been reported to enhance or slow degradation, varying from study to study. These variations are likely associated with the type and concentrations of the humic material. $^{\cdot}OH$ radicals seem to be the primary photosensitizer responsible for degrading this pollutant (De Laurentiis et al., 2012; Challis et al., 2014).

Secondly, carbamazepine is also poorly attached onto sludge. Its water-to-sludge distribution coefficient (log K_d) is far from the threshold at ~ 2.5-2.7 (i.e., K_d > 300 – 500 L kg^{-1}) which is generally considered as the minimum for significant sorption onto sludge (Ternes et al., 2004a; Joss et al., 2005; Luo et al., 2014). The water-to-soil distribution coefficient, on the other hand, is higher and sorption to soil may be considered relatively moderate.

The octanol-water partition constant, K_{ow}, which is usually used as a measure of a substance's hydrophobicity, is among the few chemical properties for which there is experimental data on carbamazepine's metabolites. From this property it is presumed that carbamazepine and some of its metabolites (most notably CBZ-EP and CBZ-2OH) have a moderate hydrophobicity. One major consequence of this particularity is that these compounds potentially may be taken up by plants: on one hand, the mild lipophilicity allows them to move across the walls of roots cells (without being irreversibly bound to them) while, on the other, they are also not too hydrophobic and are sufficiently water soluble to be transported through cell fluids. In fact it, is generally considered that contaminants with log K_{ow} between 0.5 and 3.5 are generally able to move inside plants. Conversely, compounds with log K_{ow} out of this range are either too hydrophilic or too hydrophobic to be able to easily move in and out between aqueous and lipidic media, therefore being restricted to one type of environment with a reduced mobility (Dietz and Schnoor, 2001; Tsao, 2003; Pilon-Smits, 2005).

The ionization constants (pKa) of carbamazepine and its metabolites are all very high. Therefore, these substances are expected to remain neutral and largely insensitive to pH conditions of the media.

Volatily of carbamazepine (as measured by Henry's Law constant) is well below the value of ~ $8x10^{-5}$ atm m^3 mol^{-1} (corresponding to an air-water partition coefficient (K_{aw}) of $3x10^{-3}$) which is considered the threshold for volatilization. Therefore, this physical process is not expected to be relevant in the environmental fate of carbamazepine or as a contribution to its elimination in WWTPs (Larsen et al., 2004; Hörsing et al., 2011). Thus, given the anticipated low tendency of carbamazepine to move to other compartments it can be predicted that the bulk of carbamazepine remains associated with the aqueous phase.

4. REMOVAL OF CARBAMAZEPINE IN CONVENTIONAL WWTPS

Municipal WWTPs normally receive wastewater that contains a lot of different trace pollutant compounds (both of synthetic and natural origins), which conventional treatment technologies have not been specifically designed for. The degree to which such pollutants are removed varies from near completion to almost none. In fact, the treatment processes in municipal WWTPs are designed to remove bulk constituents of wastewater, such as suspended solids, biodegradable organic matter, pathogens and nutrients, by physical, chemical and biological processes available along the consecutive stages of a conventional treatment. These conventional WWTPs typically comprise three or four stages of treatment, with different biological and physicochemical processes available for each treatment stage (Figure 4).

Given the low biological activity at preliminary and primary treatments of wastewaters, any micropollutant removal here will rely on both the tendency of the individual substances to sorb to solids (primary sludge) and the degree of suspended solids removal in the primary sedimentation tank (Carballa et al., 2004; Ternes et al., 2004a; Jones et al., 2005; Zhang et al., 2008; Zorita et al., 2009; Monteiro and Boxall, 2010; Verlicchi et al., 2012; Luo et al., 2014; Blair et al., 2015). Usually, there is little change in dissolved polar organics during screening or primary sedimentation, so little to no loss of polar pharmaceuticals may be expected at these initial stages. In general, elimination of any compound by sorption to sludge is considered relevant only when the log K_d for that compound is higher than ~ 2.5 – 2.7 (i.e., $K_d > 300 - 500$ L kg^{-1}) (Ternes et al., 2004c; Joss et al., 2005; Mohapatra et al., 2014; Verlicchi et al., 2015). That is far from being the case for carbamazepine, which has log Kd in the range of 1.3 for primary sludge (Table 2). The removal of organic micropollutants in these stages may also be affected by factors such as pH, retention time, temperature, and amount and type of solids present in the wastewater (Ternes et al., 2004c; Joss et al., 2005; Aga, 2008; Carballa et al., 2008; Verlicchi et al., 2012; Luo et al., 2014; Mohapatra et al., 2014; Verlicchi and Zambello, 2015; Blair et al., 2015).

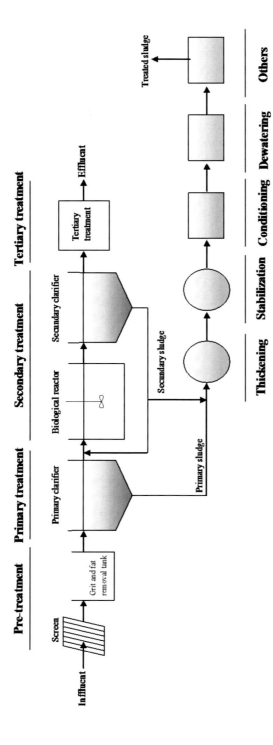

Figure 4. Diagram of a conventional wastewater treatment plant (adapted from Tchobanoglous et al. (2003)).

In some cases, not only removal of micropollutants is negligible at these stages but a release of additional amounts of contaminant may even occur during treatment, which can result from the presence in the raw influent of conjugate substances (i.e., metabolites of pharmaceuticals) that upon cleavage may produce the respective parent compounds (Ternes, 1998; Carballa et al., 2004; Zhang et al., 2008; Zorita et al., 2009; Evgenidou et al., 2015; Blair et al., 2015). Such is the case with carbamazepine, as frequently removal efficiencies of this pharmaceutical in WWTPs are reported to be negative, corresponding to the observation that its concentration in the treated WWTP effluent is higher than the concentration entering the WWTP in the raw influent, due to parent carbamazepine being regenerated by cleavage of its glucuronide conjugates (Leclercq et al., 2009; Bahlmann et al., 2014).

Activated sludge (as used in several technologies) is the most common type of secondary (biological) treatment used in conventional WWTPs. Removal of pharmaceuticals in this type of treatment may occur by the same mechanisms as other organic micropollutants do, which include sorption to and removal in secondary sludge, chemical degradation or transformation (such as hydrolysis or photodegradation) and biotransformation/ biodegradation (aerobic, anoxic or anaerobic) (Monteiro and Boxall, 2010; Verlicchi et al., 2012; Luo et al., 2014). In activated sludge processes, little loss by volatilization during aeration (stripping) is expected due to the typically low volatility of most pharmaceutical compounds (Larsen et al., 2004; Zhang et al., 2008; Miège et al., 2009; Caliman and Gavrilescu, 2009; Verlicchi et al., 2012; Luo et al., 2014; Wang and Wang, 2016) Such is also the case of carbamazepine (Table 2) whose Henry coefficient is well below the value of $\sim 8 \times 10^{-5}$ atm m^3 mol^{-1} ($K_{aw} \sim 3 \times 10^{-3}$) which is considered the threshold for significant air stripping in a bioreactor with fine bubble aeration (Larsen et al., 2004; POSEIDON, 2006; Hörsing et al., 2011). Since WWTPs are usually operated under an open environment, wastewater is exposed to direct sunlight, especially during summer. Even though sunlight may to some extent be blocked by wastewater's turbidity, exposure to sunlight irradiation may be significant for the top layer of the liquid as well as when wastewater passes the secondary clarifiers. Therefore, some contaminants may be affected by phototransformation. According to the literature (Zhang et al., 2008; Leclercq et al., 2009; Kosjek et al., 2009; Donner et al., 2013) carbamazepine can be photolysed under sunlight irradiation but only at relatively low rate. A major issue with photodegradation is the possibility that, sometimes, some degradation products may exhibit a higher toxicity than the original compound (Leclercq et al., 2009; Wang and Lin, 2014; Bergheim et al., 2014).

Carbamazepine is such a case, in which direct photolysis leads to the formation of oxidative products acridine and acridone which are known to be genotoxic (Leclercq et al., 2009).

The previous processes are only secondary in importance to biodegradation processes, which for biodegradable pollutants are the major via for pollutant removal during secondary treatment. However, in the case of the well-known recalcitrant pharmaceutical carbamazepine, which is notoriously hard to biodegrade (k_{biol} < 0.2 L g_{SS}^{-1} d^{-1}, see Table 2), little removal is obtained through these biological means. The other removal process that may have some relevance during secondary stage treatment is sorption to suspended particles and to sludge. Also in this case, carbamazepine properties (log K_d = 0.08-0.09, Table 2) do not favor these processes. Therefore, the prospects for removal of carbamazepine during secondary treatment are very low and it is expected that most of the carbamazepine entering the WWTP will leave untreated in the effluent after its secondary stage.

On the other hand, there is a possibility that carbamazepine and some of its metabolites which are present in the form glucuronide conjugates be cleaved and restore to the parent compounds, promoted by the β-glucuronidase enzyme present in activated sludge, which actually may end up increasing the amounts of carbamazepine and accompanying metabolites instead of reducing them (Ternes et al., 1999; Gomes et al., 2009; Bahlmann et al., 2014; Evgenidou et al., 2015).

Carbamazepine removal at this stage may also be affected by environmental conditions (e.g., temperature, redox conditions), type of secondary treatment (e.g., activated sludge, trickling filters, rotating biological contactors, aerated lagoons), characteristics of the biomass and operation parameters (e.g., hydraulic retention time, solid retention time, stirring and aeration conditions) (Vieno et al., 2007; Aga, 2008; Verlicchi et al., 2012; Luo et al., 2014).

Pollutants remaining in the wastewater after primary and secondary treatment may be eliminated by tertiary or advanced treatments. However, in most countries only a reduced number of WWTPs include these adaptations due to economic limitations.

In regard to the fate of carbamazepine in sludges, it is relevant to consider that primary and secondary sludge are also subjected to several stages of treatment, with different biological and physicochemical processes available for each treatment stage (Figure 4). The treatment of the sludge has the aim of increasing and stabilizing the solid organic content and reducing pathogens. As result of treatment, the water and organic content should be considerably reduced, and the processed solids should be suitable for reuse (e.g., application in soils) or final disposal (e.g., landfills, incineration). Sludge stabilization and conditioning involve changes which could affect solid partitioning, degradation, adsorption of pharmaceuticals onto sludge matrices. Sludge chemical composition may change, resulting in different adsorption behavior of compounds. This was observed by Miao et al. (2005) for carbamazepine, whose concentration increased from untreated to treated (digested and thermally dried) sludge, from 69 to 258 ng/$g_{dry\ matter}$. Nevertheless, carbamazepine is generally negligibly retained on sludges.

In summary, pollutants are subjected in WWTPs to a variety of phenomena (dispersion, dilution, partition, sorption, biodegradation and abiotic transformation) contributing to their elimination or transfer to solid phase, thereby lowering their concentration in the aqueous medium (the total removal during treatment generally refers to the losses of a parent compound contributed by all of those different processes). However, both carbamazepine and its most important metabolites seem to be considerably resistant to any of these processes, thereby exhibiting a recalcitrant behavior towards WWTP treatment that stands out in most monitoring studies of conventional plants.

Typical carbamazepine and some its metabolites loads in wastewaters and their removal by conventional treatment are presented in Table 3, which is illustrative of the inadequacy of conventional WWTPs to deal with these pollutants.

Carbamazepine and several of its metabolites are frequently present in influents entering WWTPs at concentration levels in the µg L^{-1} – ng L^{-1} range (Table 3). Carbamazepine is very persistent and little to no degradation or retention takes place in WWTPs during conventional wastewater treatment, and as result it exits in the effluent in almost the same amount as it entered the WWTP. Frequently, carbamazepine concentrations are reported to be even higher after wastewater treatment, resulting in the negative (< 0%) removal efficiencies that are reported by several authors and presented in Table 3. This outcome can be explained by several effects (Göbel et al., 2007; Zhang et al., 2008; Leclercq et al., 2009; Monteiro and Boxall, 2010; Ort et al., 2010; Verlicchi et al., 2012; Salgado et al., 2012; Kumar et al., 2012b; Bahlmann et al., 2014; Rodayan et al., 2014; Evgenidou et al., 2015; Blair et al., 2015). The main cause may be the occurrence of a cleavage of the conjugate carbamazepine-N-glucuronide with the production of the parent carbamazepine during to biological treatment. In addition, carbamazepine may be released from faecal particles as the faeces are broken down and carbamazepine is redissolved. For some pharmaceuticals desorption may also occur from the return activated sludge during the secondary treatment process, but in the case of carbamazepine this effect should represent only a minor contribution as its adsorption to sludge is generally considered negligible. Ultimately, the effect may also be overestimated in result of incorrect mass balances that do not properly address the daily concentration fluctuations and the fluid dynamics of the WWTP.

CBZ-DiOH, CBZ-2-OH, CBZ-3-OH, CBZ-EP and CBZ-10-OH are the main metabolites of carbamazepine that have been detected in several wastewaters worldwide (Table 3). In some cases, the concentrations of the metabolites even exceed the concentration of the parent compound (Table 3), in particular the metabolite CBZ-DiOH, which is the metabolite that is typically detected in higher concentrations in WWTP influents. All these above mentioned metabolites exhibit high persistence during conventional wastewater treatment (Miao and Metcalfe, 2003; Miao et al., 2005; Zhao and Metcalfe, 2008; Leclercq et al., 2009; Bahlmann et al., 2014). These metabolites can also be found in the WWTP influents in the form of glucuronide conjugates, which, like in the case of carbamazepine, also have the potential for regenerating back to the original metabolite form upon cleavage of the conjugates during treatment (with consequent observation of negative removals of those metabolites). In fact two types of glucuronide conjugates may originate from carbamazepine and its different metabolites: N-glucuronides, which occur with carbamazepine or CBZ-EP; and O-glucuronides, which occur in glucuronide conjugation with CBZ-DiOH, CBZ-2-OH, CBZ-3-OH or CBZ-10-OH. The enzyme β-glucuronidase (provided by *E. coli* from faeces and also present in activated sludge) promotes the degradation of O-glucuronides during wastewater treatment (Ternes et al., 1999; Gomes et al., 2009). On the other hand, N-glucuronides are not so prone to cleavage by β-glucuronidase (Richter et al., 1978) but, nevertheless, cleavage still occurs to a significant extent even in these cases (Bahlmann et al., 2014; Evgenidou et al., 2015).

Acridine and acridone are other frequent transformation products of carbamazepine. These two compounds, which are known to be genotoxic, are important products of carbamazepine oxidation, especially through direct photolysis under UV radiation (Leclercq et al., 2009; Kosjek et al., 2009; Donner et al., 2013).

Table 3. Influent and effluent concentrations of carbamazepine and some of its metabolites and their removal efficiency in WWTPs
(values inside brackets are average values)

Compound	Influent (µg L^{-1})	Effluent (µg L^{-1})	Removal (%)	Reference
CBZ	0.2-1.9 a	0.1–1.7 a	<0–50	(Metcalfe et al., 2003)
	(0.3689)	(0.4262)	<0	(Miao and Metcalfe, 2003)
	(0.356)	(0.251)	-	(Miao et al., 2005)
	0.12–0.31 a	0.11–0.23 a	-	(Gómez et al., 2007)
	0.16-0.82 (0.35)	0.29-2.44 (0.72)	< 0	(Vieno et al., 2007)
	0.0248–0.0509a	0.0337–0.1112a	< 0	(Spongberg and Witter, 2008)
	0.208–0.416 b	0.112–0.258 b	-10–73	(Leclercq et al., 2009)
	(0.757)	(0.713)	5.8	(Lajeunesse et al., 2012)
	0.071–1.30 a	-	-	(Writer et al., 2013)
	(1.9)	(2)	<0	(Bahlmann et al., 2014)
	-	0.43–2.76 (1.01)	-	(Gracia-Lor et al., 2014)
	-	BQL–5.811	-21–0	(Hapeshi et al., 2015)
	(0.230)	(0.166)	28	(Aymerich et al., 2016)
	(0.650)	(0.316)	51	(Petrie et al., 2016)
	0.240–0.750 a	0.290–0.770 a	<0–13	(Subedi et al., 2017)
CBZ-EP	(0.0472)	(0.0523)	<0	(Miao and Metcalfe, 2003)
	(0.0392)	(0.0191)	-	(Miao et al., 2005)
	0.3–0.5 (0.35)	<0.07–0.3 (0.16)	-	(Gómez et al., 2007)
	ND–0.026 b	<0.052–0.029 b	-	(Leclercq et al., 2009)
	(0.055)	(0.040)	27	(Aymerich et al., 2016)
	(0.036)	(0.042)	-17	(Petrie et al., 2016)
CBZ-2 OH	(0.121)	(0.1323)	<0	(Miao and Metcalfe, 2003)
	(0.059)	(0.0704)	<0	(Miao et al., 2005)
	ND–0.037 b	<0.005–0.048 b	-	(Leclercq et al., 2009)
	(0.508)	(0.622)	<0	(Aymerich et al., 2016)
CBZ-3 OH	(0.0948)	(0.1015)	<0	(Miao and Metcalfe, 2003)
	(0.0554)	(0.0692)	<0	(Miao et al., 2005)
CBZ-10 OH	(0.0085)	(0.0093)	<0	(Miao and Metcalfe, 2003)
	(0.0222)	(0.0325)	<0	(Miao et al., 2005)
	ND–1.065 b	<0.075–1.170 b	<0	(Leclercq et al., 2009)
	< 0.010–1.9	-	-	(Writer et al., 2013)
CBZ-DiOH	(1.5717)	(1.325)	-	(Miao and Metcalfe, 2003)
	(1.0012)	(1.0812)	<0	(Miao et al., 2005)
	0.325–1.415	0.311–1.50	<0	(Leclercq et al., 2009)
	<0.010–0.260	-	-	(Writer et al., 2013)
	-	0.55–6.85 (1.76)	-	(Gracia-Lor et al., 2014)
	(0.0185)	(0.103)	-457	(Petrie et al., 2016)
Acridine (AI)	ND–0.018 b	<0.0057–0.026b	-	(Leclercq et al., 2009)
Acridone (AO)	ND–0.019 b	ND–0.023 b	-	(Leclercq et al., 2009)

a: concentrations range detected in a single WWTP; b: mean concentration ranges detected in a set of WWTPs; ND: not detected.

In light of the available data, of which Table 3 presents a sample, the limitations of conventional WWTPs to deal with contamination by carbamazepine and its metabolites is very clear. Such inefficiency to remove carbamazepine adds to a general inefficiency of conventional WWTPs in regard to many other organic micropollutants such as other pharmaceuticals, pesticides, polyaromatic hydrocarbons, etc. Aiming to improve the efficiency of WWTPs in removing some of these types of pollutants, optimization of conventional wastewater treatment processes and WWTPs operation parameters has already been attempted but that usually has only allowed for modest improvements. In addition several advanced treatment technologies have also been evaluated which in some cases could significantly enhance pollutants removal efficiencies. However, some of these advanced technologies incur in significant cost to implement and operate, which limits their economically viability and hinders their wide adoption, sometimes limiting them to only some niches of industrial wastewaters (Fent et al., 2006).

Even though no single wastewater treatment technology that is effective for micropollutants cleanup has yet been found and generally adopted, the issue of emergent pollutants such as pharmaceuticals has become one of the top topics in environmental science over the last years and the need for adequate regulations aiming at mitigating this type of contaminants have been raised several times by experts (Robinson et al., 2007; Bolong et al., 2009). In fact, greater awareness to this problem has been arising as environmental agencies worldwide have been electing these new substances as priority pollutants and requiring new environmental risk assessments to be carried out as part of the process of approving new substances for public use (Kot-Wasik et al., 2007). In this context, it is conceivable that wastewater treatment requirements become more stringent in the future in terms of setting some limits to the concentrations of many of these substances in the treated effluents of WWTPs. Consequently, given the general inefficiency of conventional treatments in regard to these pollutants, there is a growing need for alternative/complementary wastewater treatment processes with higher efficiencies at reasonable costs of operation/maintenance that are especially suited for removing this range of contaminants of which carbamazepine is a prominent representative.

5. Alternative/Complementary Removal Technologies in WWTPs

Conventional wastewater treatment based on the technology of *activated sludge* is currently deemed as one of the most cost-effective wastewater treatment technologies available to date. However, if at a reasonably low cost the removal of bulk pollutants is attained with high efficiencies through this technology, contrarily in regard to organic micropollutants, such as pharmaceutical residues, it usually only attains partial removal of most such compounds like carbamazepine. Thus, it is quite evident that more advanced technologies must complement (or, in some specific cases, substitute) conventional treatment in order to fulfill more stringent WWTP effluent quality goals or to comply with requirements for municipal wastewater reuse.

Over the latest years various advanced treatment technologies have been assessed for removal of pharmaceutical compounds including carbamazepine, which my be present in wastewaters as trace pollutants. Among them adsorption processes, membrane treatment using both biological (membrane bioreactors) and non-biological processes (reversed osmosis, ultrafiltration, nanofiltration), and advanced oxidation processes (AOP) are the technologies that have been more extensively studied, both in lab experiments and at pilot scale. Even if some of these technologies achieve very high efficiencies, the excessive cost of implementation as well as of operation and maintenance is the major drawback holding back the adoption of most of these currently available advanced treatment technologies. As a more economic alternative, technologies that are based on the water depurating capabilities of some aquatic plants, among which constructed wetlands systems (CWS) are one of the most commonplace, for the removal of pharmaceuticals residues has been increasingly explored in recent years. In fact, these systems are becoming an option for secondary wastewater treatment systems or as treatment units for polishing secondary effluent from WWTPs. In addition to low cost, the conveniences of simple operation and maintenance (thereby not requiring highly skilled labour), environmental friendliness and good integration with the landscape (thereby providing better aesthetics and general public acceptance) are some of their most attractive characteristics.

In Table 4 a short overview is presented of some of the most frequently studied advanced treatment processes as well as of constructed wetland systems, along with some of the carbamazepine removal efficiencies that are to be expected from typical case studies for each of those technologies.

Table 4. Carbamazepine removal efficiencies attained in illustrative cases of studies on advanced treatment processes and on constructed wetland systems

Treatment Process	Assays conditions	Removal efficiency (%)	References
Adsorption processes			
• Carbonaceus materials			
GAC	Carbon column 1-50 mg/L	74-86	(Snyder et al., 2007)
PAC	Surface water Adsrobent: 5 mg/L CBZ: 100 ng/L	~ 70	(Snyder et al., 2007)
GAC	Synthetic water Adsorbent: 10 mg/L CBZ: 500 ng/L	100	(Yu et al., 2008)
MWCNT (10-60)	Distilled water Adsorbent:1 and 2 mg, pH 7, 23°C CBZ: 2.5 mg/L	62.7-90.6	(Oleszczuk et al., 2009)
PAC (Norit SAE super)	Hospital wastewater Adsorbent: 8, 23, 43 mg/L CBZ: 0.235 µg/L	98-100	(Kovalova et al., 2013)
PAC	WWTPs effluents Adsorbent: 50 mg/L CBZ: 2.5 µg/L	90	(Altmann et al., 2014)
Filtrasorb 400	Spiked secondary treated domestic wastewater Adsorbent: 35 g/L CBZ: 0.1-10 µg/L; 100-1000 µg/L	99.7; 99.5	(Tahar et al., 2014)
Graphene	WWTPs effluents CBZ: 10 mg/L	97 (62 d)	(Rizzo et al., 2015)
• Clay-based materials			
Expanded clay (LECA)	Pure water (PW) and WWTPs effluents (WW) A solid to liquid ratio of 1.0 kg/L CBZ: 1-50 mg/L	60– 95 PW 51 – 93 WW (144 h)	(Dordio et al., 2009)
Modified smectites (montmorillonite)	Pure water Adsorbents: cation-exchanged with K^+, Ca^{2+}, NH_4^+, TMA, TMPA and HDTMA CBZ: 50-5000 µg/L		(Zhang et al., 2010)

Table 4. (Continued)

Treatment Process		Assays conditions	Removal efficiency (%)	References
	Modified bentonite	Pure water Adsorbents: organo-bentonites and organo-bentonites modified with metals; 20g/L CBZ: 14 mg/L	62-88	(Rivera-Jimenez et al., 2011)
	Expanded clay (Filtralite HC)	Spiked secondary treated domestic wastewater Adsorbent: 35 g/L CBZ: 0.1-10 μg/L; 100-1000 μg/L	67.4; 62.2	(Tahar et al., 2014)
• Zeolites				
	Y	Wastewater	100	(Martucci et al., 2012)
	Clinoptinolite	Spiked secondary treated domestic wastewater Adsorbent: 35 g/L CBZ: 0.1-10 μg/L; 100-1000 μg/L	23.3; 59.6	(Tahar et al., 2014)
• Agricultural wastes and by products				
	Cork (granulated)	Pure water (PW) and WWTPs effluents (WW) Solid to liquid ratio: 0.1 kg/L CBZ. 1-35 mg/L	68-88 PW 63 WW (144 h)	(Dordio et al., 2011)
Advanced Oxidation Processes (AOP)				
• Fenton and photo-Fenton				
		Wastewater Fe: 5 and 20 mg/L H_2O_2: 50 mg/L, pH 3, solar UV radiation (<400 nm) CBZ: 5 and 100 μg/L	100 (150 min)	(Klamerth et al., 2010)
		Wastewater Fe^{2+}: 0.016 mM, room temperature, pH 3 H_2O_2:0.8 mM CBZ: 100 μg/L	>90 (180 min)	(Mohapatra et al., 2013)
		Ultrapure water Fe^{2+}: 0.1 mM, Persulphate: 0.2 mM, 25°C, pH 8.4, CBZ: 50 μM	100 (30 min)	(Ahmed and Chiron, 2014)

Treatment Process	Assays conditions	Removal efficiency (%)	References
	Ultrapure water Fe_3O_4: 1.0 g/L, 23°C, pH 7.0 H_2O_2:100 mM CBZ: 60.35 μM	100 (120 min)	(Sun et al., 2014)
• Ozonation (O_3)			
	Raw river water O_3: 1.5–2 mg/L CBZ:	100 (20 min)	(Hua et al., 2006)
	Wastewater O_3: 3 mg/L CBZ: 2.3-33.3 ng/L	> 81 (27 min)	(Nakada et al., 2007)
	Water O_3: 0.22 mM, pH 3, 7, 25°C CBZ: 15 mg/L	100	(Rosal et al., 2008)
	Natural water/ ultrapure water O_3: 80 mM, pH 3,9, 20°C CBZ: 50 μM	20-30 (20 min)	(Real et al., 2009)
	Ultrapure water O_3: 3.5 mg/L, pH 6,7,8,15°C CBZ: 10 mg/L	100 (60 min)	(Antoniou and Andersen, 2012)
	Ultrapure water O_3: 1.2 g/L pH 7.0 CBZ: 11 mg/L	100 (30 min)	(Palo et al., 2012)
	Hospital wastewater O_3:4.2, 5.8, 7 mg/L	> 99	(Kovalova et al., 2013)
	Drinking water O_3: 2 mg/L, pH 7.3 CBZ: 278 μg/L	100 (10 min)	(Tootchi et al., 2013)
• TiO₂ photocatalysis			
TiO₂/Artificial sunlight	Lake water with 0.5 mg/L NOM TiO_2: 100 mg/L	75 (9 min)	(Doll and Frimmel, 2005)
TiO2,/solar UV	Wastewater UV intensity: 30 W/m^2 CBZ: 100 μg/L	100 (120 min)	(Miranda-García et al., 2011)
• UV and UV/Hydrogen peroxide treatment			
UV/ H_2O_2	Surface water UVntensity: 853 mJ/cm^2 H_2O_2: 10 mg/L	90	(Pereira et al., 2007)
UV	Distilled water UV lamp 690 W CBZ: 100 μg/L	93 (10 min)	(Kosjek et al., 2009)

Table 4. (Continued)

Treatment Process	Assays conditions	Removal efficiency (%)	References
UV/ H_2O_2	Wastewater UV intensity: 2768 mJ/cm²; room temperature, pH 6.5 H_2O_2: 1.72 g/L. CBZ: ~95 ng/L	100 (15 min)	(Kim et al., 2009)
UV/H_2O_2	Wastewater UV intensity: 300 to 700 mJ/cm², 18°C H_2O_2: 2, 5, 10, 15 and 20 mg/L CBZ: 210 and 320 ng/L	10 to 90 (6 to 20 min)	(Rosario-Ortiz et al., 2010)
UV/ H_2O_2	Distilled deionized water UV 254 nm, 25°C, pH 5 H_2O_2:11 mM CBZ: 1 mg/L	< 40 (30 min)	(Giri et al., 2010)
UV/ H_2O_2	Wastewater UV intensity: 550 w/m², 17°C, pH 2.5 H_2O_2: 50 mg/L CBZ: 263 ng/L	100 (30 min)	(De la Cruz et al., 2012)
UV/O_3/H_2O_2	Deionized water UV intensity: 0–12.8 mW/cm² O_3: 0–1.2 mg/L H_2O_2: 0–34 mg/L	6.6-98	(Im et al., 2012)
UV	Hospital wastewater UV intensity:88-7200 J/m²	1	(Kovalova et al., 2013)
UV/ H_2O_2	Deionized water UV intensity: 153 mM/cm², 25°C, pH 3.0 H_2O_2: 5 mM, CBZ: 21.16 µM	> 95 (45 min)	(Deng et al., 2013)
UV/ H_2O_2	Ultrapure water UV intensity: 500 mJ/cm²; pH 6.5 H_2O_2: 10 mg/L CBZ: 1.0 µg/L	> 99	(Wols et al., 2014)
Membrane processes			
• Membrane bioreactor (MBR)			
	Wastewater SRT:10 d	0	(Clara et al., 2004a)
	Wastewater SRT: 11 d	11	(Kreuzinger et al., 2004)

Treatment Process	Assays conditions	Removal efficiency (%)	References
	Synthetic wastewater Lab-scale Polyvinylidene fluoride HF MA: 0.2 m²; Pore size: 0.4 μm HRT: 1 d or 3 d; MLSS: 2.3-4.6 g/L	minor	(Bo et al., 2009)
	Hospital effluent Full-scale 5 Kubota EK 400 flat sheet Q: 130 m/d	<20	(Beier et al., 2011)
	Synthetic wastewater Lab-scale submerged HF UF module MA: 0.047m²; Pore size: 0.04 μm SRT:70 d; HRT: 24 h MLSS: 8.6-10 g/L	13.4 ± 4.3	(Tadkaew et al., 2011)
	Hospital effluent Pilot-scale Submerged PES UF flat sheet Area: 7 m²; Pore size: 38 nm SRT: 30-50 d MLSS: 2 g/L	-6	(Kovalova et al., 2012)
	Raw wastewater Full-scale HF (Koch Puron); MA:235 m²; Pore size:0.1-0.2 μm SRT: 10-15 d; HRT: 1 d MLSS: 7.5-8.5 g/L	24	(Trinh et al., 2012)
	Wastewater	39	(Wijekoon et al., 2015)
	Wastewater	< 10	(González-Pérez et al., 2016)
• Non biological membrane processes			
Nanofiltration	Water Pilot scale (N90) CBZ: 100-700 ng/L	> 95	(Bellona et al., 2008)
Osmose reverse	Water Pilot scale (TME 10) CBZ: 100-700 ng/L	> 95	(Bellona et al., 2008)
Osmose reverse	Water Pilot scale (TFC-HR) CBZ: 100-700 ng/L	> 95	(Bellona et al., 2008)

Table 4. (Continued)

Treatment Process	Assays conditions	Removal efficiency (%)	References
Osmose reverse	Water Pilot scale (ESPAZ) CBZ: 100-700 ng/L	> 95	(Bellona et al., 2008)
Nanofiltration	Drinking water Full scale (NF 90-400) CBZ: 8.7-166.5 ng/L	> 98	(Radjenovic et al., 2008)
Osmose Reverse	Drinking water Full scale (BW 30 LE-440) CBZ: 8.7-166.5 ng/L	> 98	(Radjenovic et al., 2008)
Nanofiltration	WWTP effluent Flat-sheet, Area: 3.5 m^2; TMP: 0.3 or 0.7 bar	minor	(Röhricht et al., 2009)
Nanofiltration	Water Pilot scale (Desal HL) CBZ: 2 µg/L	64-84	(Verliefde et al., 2009)
Nanofiltration	Water Lab scale NF (Filmtec NF 200 and NF 90) CBZ: 8-17 µg/L	~ 80 (NF 200) ~ 90 (NF 90)	(Yangali-Quintanilla et al., 2011)
Constructed wetlands systems			
Horizontal subsurface flow (*pilot*)	Wastewater Gravel/ *Phragmites australis*	26 (deep) 16 (shallow)	(Matamoros et al., 2005)
Horizontal subsurface flow (*pilot*)	Wastewater Gravel/ *Phragmites australis*	16	(Matamoros and Bayona, 2006)
Vertical subsurface flow (*pilot*)	Wastewater Gravel/ *Phragmites australis*	26	(Matamoros et al., 2007)
Surface flow (*full*)	Wastewater *Typha* spp. + *Phragmites australis*	30-47	(Matamoros et al., 2008)
Surface flow (*pilot*)	Wastewater *Acorus* + *Typha* spp.	65	(Park et al., 2009)
Horizontal subsurface flow (*full*)	Wastewater *Phragmites australis*	38	(Matamoros et al., 2009)
Vertical Subsurface Flow (*microcosms*)	Wastewater Expanded clay/*Typha* spp	88 (winter) 97 (summer)	(Dordio et al., 2010)
Horizontal subsurface flow (*mesocosms*)	Wastewater Gravel/*Phragmites australis* or *Typha angustifolia*	22-50	(Hijosa-Valsero et al., 2010)

Treatment Process		Assays conditions	Removal efficiency (%)	References
	Horizontal subsurface flow *(mesocosms)*	Wastewater Gravel/*Typha angustifolia*	27	(Zhang et al., 2011)
	Horizontal subsurface flow *(mesocosms)*	Wastewater Gravel/*Typha angustifolia*	27	(Zhang et al., 2012)
	Horizontal subsurface flow *(mesocosms)*	Wastewater Gravel/*Phragmites australis* or *Typha angustifolia*	n.r.-70	(Reyes-Contreras et al., 2012)
	Surface flow *(mesocosms)*	Wastewater *Phragmites australis/ Typha angustifolia*	n.r.-95	(Reyes-Contreras et al., 2012)
	Subsurface flow *(microcosms)*	Wastewater Ceramsite and gravel/*Cyperus alternifolius*	64	(Yan et al., 2016)

CBZ: carbamazepine; GAC: granular activated carbon; MA: membrane area; MWCNT: multiwalled carbon canotubes; PAC: powdered activated carbon.

The data reported in Table 4 refers to a wide variety of study types, spanning lab, pilot or full scale systems and obtained on real media (water or wastewater) as well as on synthetic model media. Therefore, sometimes comparisons of results reported by different researchers for the same type of technology can not be established in a straightforward manner.

However, the sample of studies presented in Table 4 clearly illustrates how application of advanced treatment processes downstream of conventional processes can in some cases significantly enhance the removal of carbamazepine. In fact, advanced technologies such as adsorption processes, advanced oxidation processes and membrane processes, seem to be promising alternatives for removal recalcitrant pollutants such carbamazepine in respect to the high efficiencies that have been attained in many cases.

Adsorption processes have been found to be relatively effective for the removal of organic micropollutants from water and wastewater. These processes are in general superior to other technologies for water decontamination in terms of the flexibility and simplicity of design, ease of operation and insensitivity to toxic pollutants. Treatment by adsorption also does not result in the formation of harmful substances. Its cost of implementation, however, is primarily related with the cost of the adsorbents used and of their regeneration.

Activated carbon is one of the oldest, most popular and widely used adsorbents. It has long been used in water and wastewater treatment, being a recognised technology for the removal of both natural and synthetic organic contaminants and, thus, researchers have explored the possibility of using this process for removing emerging pollutants including carbamazepine (Table 4).

Almost any carbonaceous material may be used as a precursor for the preparation of activated carbons, the main requirement being that it possesses a high carbon content.

Granular activated carbon can be used in conventional filters, providing both adsorption and filtration, and can be applied following conventional activated sludge treatment. The biggest barrier to the general use of activated carbon is its cost and the difficulties associated with regeneration (Derbyshire et al., 2001; Chen et al., 2011; Tahar et al., 2013). In general, activated carbon is quite expensive and the higher the quality the greater the cost. The use of carbons based on relatively expensive starting materials is unjustified for most pollution control applications (Streat et al., 1995). Also, both chemical and thermal regeneration of spent carbon is expensive, impractical on a large scale and produces additional effluent and results in considerable loss of the adsorbent. Therefore, much attention has been given in recent years to the research of low cost and easily available natural materials such as clays or zeolites, certain agricultural wastes s and other industrial wastes and by-products (Table 4). Some of these low cost materials have shown significantly high removal capacities for a variety of organic micropollutants, which presents an interest prospect for the application of sorption processes as cost-effective water and wastewater treatment options for dealing with this class of contaminants.

Conventional chemical oxidation is an important treatment process for both water and wastewater that is commonly used for providing disinfection. Notably, these reactions also have the potential to attain transformation (partial oxidation) or complete elimination of organic micropollutants such as carbamazepine. Thus, substantial research effort is being put into optimizing and enhancing their effects using advanced oxidation processes (AOPs), which has lately been emerging as an important class of wastewater treatment technologies (Table 4).

AOPs involve the generation and use of powerful oxidizing agents leading to oxidation and mineralization of organic matter with enhanced reaction rate constants, although also being characterized by a lack of selectivity of attack (Rivera-Utrilla et al., 2013).

These processes are characterized and differentiated by the methods of producing oxidizing agents, which involve combinations of chemical agents (e.g., ozone (O_3), hydrogen peroxide (H_2O_2), transition metals, and metal oxides) and auxiliary energy sources (e.g., ultraviolet-visible (UV-Vis) radiation, electronic current, γ-radiation, and ultrasound). Because of these differences in reagent and equipment requirements, the cost of generating the oxidizing agents varies greatly for different AOPs.

Examples of AOPs that have been used and evaluated (mainly at a bench scale, but many of the processes are being developed at a pilot-scale as well) include O_3/H_2O_2, O_3/UV, $O_3/H_2O_2/UV$, H_2O_2/UV, Fenton (Fe^{2+}/H_2O_2), photo- and electro-Fenton, chelating agent assisted Fenton/photo-Fenton, heterogeneous photo-oxidation using titanium dioxide ($TiO_2/h\upsilon$), γ-radiolysis, and sonolysis (Rivera-Utrilla et al., 2013; Luo et al., 2014; Mohapatra et al., 2014; Ganzenko et al., 2014; Wang and Wang, 2016). This diversity of techniques is responsible for the versatility of AOPs (Rivera-Utrilla et al., 2013; Luo et al., 2014; Mohapatra et al., 2014) that facilitates the compliance with specific treatment requirements.

Some of the advantages of AOPs include the possibility of complete mineralization of organic contaminants, or production of less harmful and more biodegradable by-products, and ability to handle fluctuating wastewater flow rates and compositions (Zhou and Smith, 2001). However, most studies do not include information on the by-products formed during the application AOPs or any information related to the activity of the by-products. Therefore, these processes should be carefully monitored and ecotoxicological investigations should be conducted to investigate the formation of potentially toxic transformation products (Fatta-Kassinos et al., 2011; Mohapatra et al., 2013; Ganzenko et al., 2014).

In addition, materials and equipment costs as well as energy requirements and efficiency must be taken into account when assessing the overall performance of AOPs (Ikehata et al., 2006).

Among the different AOPs studied for the degradation of carbamazepine from wastewater, it was observed that the ozone based techniques (O_3, O_3/H_2O_2, O_3/UV) and UV/H_2O_2 process have gained the widest application (Table 4). The UV/H_2O_2 process has a distinct advantage because of its simplicity. The only chemical required is H_2O_2, which is easily available, easily stored and precisely fed according to the process demand. Thus, the UV/H_2O_2 process is well suited to small systems that required no additional equipment or material of construction, minimum maintenance, and intermittent operation, or both. The O_3/UV process is considered less favourable than the O_3/H_2O_2 and UV/H_2O_2 processes. It has been reported that the rate of ozone consumption per unit volume in case of O_3/UV process can be so high that mass transfer limited regime for ozone absorption is established thus resulting in a decrease of quantum efficiencies and an increase of operating cost.

In regard to the use of membrane processes for the removal of pharmaceuticals from contaminated water, a diversity of membrane system types (including microfiltration, ultrafiltration, nanofiltration, reverse osmosis, electro dialysis reversal, membrane bioreactors and combinations of membranes in series) have already been tested either at pilot or full scale (Bolong et al., 2009; Luo et al., 2014; Cincinelli et al., 2015). However, microfiltration and ultrafiltration are generally considered ineffective in removing organic micropollutants as pore sizes vary from 100-1000 times larger than this type of contaminants, thus allowing them to slip through the membranes (Deegan et al., 2011).

Reverse osmosis and nanofiltration are mostly assessed as promising alternatives for eliminating micropollutants including pharmaceuticals and these membrane technologies have been evaluated and employed in tertiary wastewater treatment for wastewater reclamation and reuse (Park et al., 2004; Yoon et al., 2006; Snyder et al., 2007; Yoon et al., 2007; Acero et al., 2010; Acero et al., 2012; Siegrist and Joss, 2012; Plumlee et al., 2014) but studies concerning carbamazepine removal is still somewhat limited.

Comparatively, the nanofiltration membrane is "looser" than reverse osmosis. The latter will give, in many cases, almost complete removal, but the higher energy consumption is a less attractive feature of this option (Vedavyasan, 2000; Plumlee et al., 2014).

In addition to non-biological processes, membrane process like microfiltration or ultrafiltration may be combined with a suspended growth bioreactor in what is called the membrane bioreactor (MBR) for wastewater treatment (Melin et al., 2006; Judd, 2008; Li et al., 2014a). Thus MBRs combine biodegradation in a conventional activated sludge process with a separation step to retain sludge in the system for higher removal of micropollutants such as pharmaceuticals (Melin et al., 2006; Judd, 2008; Kovalova et al., 2012; Trinh et al., 2012; Melo-Guimaraes et al., 2013; Nguyen et al., 2013; Li et al., 2014a).

These reactors can be composed of two units: a bioreactor tank and a membrane module, but generally, these two units are combined in only one, where the membrane unit is submerged inside the bioreactor (Melin et al., 2006; Li et al., 2014a).

The separation of biology and membrane compartments allows different aeration systems and oxygen concentrations in both compartments. In the biology part, fine bubble aeration supplies oxygen for the bacteria necessary for the oxidation of substrates, while in the membrane compartment coarse bubble aeration is used to generate enough turbulence to decrease as much as possible membrane fouling and clogging, which are the major drawbacks of such processes. The membranes are in contact with the sludge but reject the sludge solids while the water permeates through the membranes. Additionally, anoxic or anaerobic biology tanks can be added for nitrogen and biological phosphorous removal.

The mechanisms involved in MBR for pharmaceuticals removal may include physical retention by membrane, biotransformation, air stripping, sorption, and photo-transformation (Larsen et al., 2004; Sipma et al., 2010; Verlicchi et al., 2012; Li et al., 2014a; González-Pérez et al., 2016). To date, studies on laboratory, pilot or full scale MBR systems have reported only negligible to very moderate removals of carbamazepine, which are comparable to those obtained with activated sludge (Table 4).

Several reviews are available where the advantages and disadvantages of the different advanced treatment technologies are discussed (Jones et al., 2005; Bolong et al., 2009; Klavarioti et al., 2009; Kummerer, 2009; Fatta-Kassinos et al., 2011; Rivera-Utrilla et al., 2013; Mohapatra et al., 2014; Ganzenko et al., 2014). In summary, it can be concluded that much higher efficiencies can generally be attainable by advanced treatment technologies, but all of these technologies have more or less specific shortcomings:

- Many of these technologies have high costs of implementation and/or operation and maintenance, and also require more expensive skilled labor;
- Efficiency may depend strongly on the type of compound;
- None of the technologies can remove all of the compounds (Rivera-Utrilla et al., 2013; Ganzenko et al., 2014);
- Will they work for new compounds in the future? (Kummerer, 2009);
- Mutagenic and toxic properties have been found for the reaction products of (photo) oxidation processes (Fatta-Kassinos et al., 2011; Michael et al., 2013; Ganzenko et al., 2014; Rizzo et al., 2015);
- Resistance in biomembrane reactors: would the enrichment of antibiotics and resistant bacteria cause increasing resistance? No information is available on this topic (Bergheim et al., 2014);
- Resistance material will not fully be retained by membranes (Kummerer, 2009);
- Requirements of energy input are higher for membrane processes.

As a more cost-efficient alternative to most advanced treatment technologies, constructed wetland systems (CWS) are being increasingly used as an option to remove organic micropollutants from wastewaters. CWS are engineered systems designed and constructed to emulate natural wetlands and to make use of the natural processes involving wetland vegetation, soils and their associated microbial assemblages in order to assist in wastewater treatment. They take advantage of many of the same processes that occur in natural wetlands, but do so within a more controlled environment (Cooper et al., 1996; Vymazal et al., 1998; Kadlec and Wallace, 2009; Dordio and Carvalho, 2013; Verlicchi and Zambello, 2014).

There is a large variety of studies highlighting the high efficiencies of these systems in removing a several different types of compounds. For this reason, this type of systems are being adopted as a tertiary treatment option in domestic wastewater treatment and, also, at least as part of the specialized wastewater treatment plants of some industries (such as chemical, dye, tannery, livestock, etc.). However, available studies specifically focusing the removal of pharmaceuticals are still relatively recent, and especially those including carbamazepine are still somewhat scarce. Notwithstanding, from available data, which have been obtained at all different system scales (microcosm, mesocosm, pilot or full scale), varied carbamazepine removal efficiencies are obtained that make it difficult to conclude on general trends of these systems performance in regard to carbamazepine treatment. This variance is certainly influenced by the rather varied options for the systems' design, namely the plant species used, the materials employed in the support matrices, the type of flow, etc. Conversely, there is enough flexibility in the systems' construction and operation that allows for ample optimization, which at best allows to reach similar efficiencies as most advanced treatment processes at a much lower cost of operation and maintenance. In the past, CWS have often been studied as "black boxes" where only influent and effluent pollutant concentrations were determined and improvements to CWS design were assessed based on a simple trial-and-error approach, without further in-depth investigations of the components characteristics and pollutant removal mechanisms being pursued. In recent years, increasingly an effort has been undertaken, as a new trend in the research on CWS, to thoroughly characterize some of the processes involved in pollutants removal in CWS, as well as to improve the understanding regarding the ways the several CWS components (solid matrix, vegetation and microorganisms) may interact with each other synergistically (Truu et al., 2009; Dordio and Carvalho, 2013; Carvalho et al., 2014; Verlicchi and Zambello, 2014; Garcia-Rodriguez et al.,

2014; Zhang et al., 2014; Li et al., 2014b). As result of the accumulated knowledge on these processes and interactions, a better guidance in the selection and optimization of the CWS components is becoming possible to refine the use of CWS for the removal of more recalcitrant pollutants such as carbamazepine.

CONCLUSION

Carbamazepine is a notorious case of a recalcitrant organic micropollutant that is frequently detected in all kinds of aqueous media, from wastewaters to natural water resources (both ground and surface water) and even in tap water. More recently it has been also detected in soils (due to application of contaminated water in irrigation or contaminated sludges as fertilizer) and inside some plants (because some species can uptake carbamazepine from contaminated water). Even more than being due to its large worldwide consumption, carbamazepine's ubiquity as a contaminant of aqueous environments and soils can mainly be attributed to its resistance to degradation. The major source of contamination can be pinpointed to wastewater treatment plants, which are generally ineffective to eliminate this pollutant. Furthermore, in addition to carbamazepine, its many metabolites that are excreted after ingestion and transformation by the human body, also largely share the parent's drug recalcitrant nature. However, these substances are much more poorly characterized as well as their effects in ecosystems and to public health. Therefore, one of the major issues concerning the ecotoxicological risks posed by contamination with carbamazepine that will need significantly more research work in the future is the effects (especially those that are chronic, due to a long-term exposure) that may be caused not only by carbamazepine but also by its main metabolites, which need an overall better characterization.

A considerable improvement of alternative/complementary water and wastewater treatment processes is a goal than needs to be pursued in general to make existing WWTPs capable of coping with emergent pollutants, as this is becoming one of the major issues of environmental science currently. In particular, carbamazepine presents a specially difficult challenge that will require significant progress in this field to be overcome.

REFERENCES

Acero, J. L.; Benitez, F. J.; Leal, A. I.; Real, F. J.; Teva, F. *J. Hazard. Mater.* **2010**, *177*, 390-398.

Acero, J. L.; Benitez, F. J.; Real, F. J.; Teva, F. *Chem. Eng. J.* **2012**, *210*, 1-8.

Aga, D. S. *Fate of Pharmaceuticals in the Environment and in Water Treatment Systems*; CRC Press: Boca Raton, FL, 2008.

Ahmed, M. M.; Chiron, S. *Water Res.* **2014**, *48*, 229-236.

Al Rajab, A. J.; Sabourin, L.; Lapen, D. R.; Topp, E. *Sci. Total Environ.* **2015**, *512–513*, 480-488.

Almeida, A.; Calisto, V.; Esteves, V. I.; Schneider, R. J.; Soares, A. M. V. M.; Figueira, E.; Freitas, R. *Aquat. Toxicol.* **2014**, *156*, 74-87.

Altmann, J.; Ruhl, A. S.; Zietzschmann, F.; Jekel, M. *Water Res.* **2014**, *55*, 185-193.

Andreozzi, R.; Marotta, R.; Pinto, G.; Pollio, A. *Water Res.* **2002**, *36*, 2869-2877.

Andreozzi, R.; Raffaele, M.; Nicklas, P. *Chemosphere* **2003**, *50*, 1319-1330.

Antoniou, M. G.; Andersen, H. R. *Environ. Technol.* **2012**, *33*, 1747-1753.

Archer, E.; Petrie, B.; Kasprzyk-Hordern, B.; Wolfaardt, G. M. *Chemosphere* **2017**.

Arnold, K. E.; Brown, A. R.; Ankley, G. T.; Sumpter, J. P. *Philos. Trans. R. Soc. B-Biol. Sci.* **2014**, *369*.

Arnold, W. A.; McNeill, K. In *Analysis, fate and removal of pharmaceuticals in the water cycle*; Petrovic, M.; Barceló, D.; Eds.; Elsevier: Amsterdam, Netherlands, 2007; pp 361-385.

Aymerich, I.; Acuña, V.; Barceló, D.; García, M. J.; Petrovic, M.; Poch, M.; Rodriguez-Mozaz, S.; Rodríguez-Roda, I.; Sabater, S.; von Schiller, D.; Corominas, L. *Water Res.* **2016**, *100*, 126-136.

Aznar, R.; Sánchez-Brunete, C.; Albero, B.; Rodríguez, J. A.; Tadeo, J. L. *Environ. Sci. Pollut. Res.* **2014**, *21*, 4772-4782.

Azuma, T.; Arima, N.; Tsukada, A.; Hirami, S.; Matsuoka, R.; Moriwake, R.; Ishiuchi, H.; Inoyama, T.; Teranishi, Y.; Yamaoka, M.; Mino, Y.; Hayashi, T.; Fujita, Y.; Masada, M. *Sci. Total Environ.* **2016**, *548–549*, 189-197.

Bahlmann, A.; Brack, W.; Schneider, R. J.; Krauss, M. *Water Res.* **2014**, *57*, 104-114.

Barra Caracciolo, A.; Topp, E.; Grenni, P. *J. Pharm. Biomed. Anal.* **2015**, *106*, 25-36.

Barron, L.; Havel, J.; Purcell, M.; Szpak, M.; Kelleher, B.; Paull, B. *Analyst* **2009**, *134*, 663-670.

Bartrons, M.; Peñuelas, J. *Trends Plant Sci.* **2017**.

Beausse, J. *TrAC Trends Anal. Chem.* **2004**, *23*, 753-761.

Behera, S. K.; Kim, H. W.; Oh, J. E.; Park, H. S. *Sci. Total Environ.* **2011**, *409*, 4351-4360.

Beier, S.; Cramer, C.; Köster, S.; Mauer, C.; Palmowski, L.; Schröder, H. F.; Pinnekamp, J. *Water Sci. Technol.* **2011**, *63*, 66.

Bellona, C.; Drewes, J. E.; Oelker, G.; Luna, J.; Filteau, G.; Amy, G. *J. Am. Water Works Assoc.* **2008**, *100*, 102-116.

Bergheim, M.; Gminski, R.; Spangenberg, B.; Debiak, M.; Burkle, A.; Mersch-Sundermann, V.; Kummerer, K.; Giere, R. *Environ. Chem.* **2014**, *11*, 431-444.

Blair, B.; Nikolaus, A.; Hedman, C.; Klaper, R.; Grundl, T. *Chemosphere* **2015**, *134*, 395-401.

Bo, L.; Urase, T.; Wang, X. *Front. Environ. Sci. Eng. China* **2009**, *3*, 236-240.

Bolong, N.; Ismail, A. F.; Salim, M. R.; Matsuura, T. *Desalination* **2009**, *239*, 229-246.

Bondarenko, S.; Gan, J.; Ernst, F.; Green, R.; Baird, J.; McCullough, M. *J. Environ. Qual.* **2012**, *41*, 1268-1274.

Boxall, A. B. A. *EMBO Rep.* **2004**, *5*, 1110-1116.

Brandão, F. P.; Rodrigues, S.; Castro, B. B.; Gonçalves, F.; Antunes, S. C.; Nunes, B. *Aquat. Toxicol.* **2013**, *144–145*, 218-229.

Cabeza, Y.; Candela, L.; Ronen, D.; Teijon, G. *J. Hazard. Mater.* **2012**, *239-240*, 32-39.

Calderón-Preciado, D.; Matamoros, V.; Savé, R.; Muñoz, P.; Biel, C.; Bayona, J. M. *Environ. Sci. Pollut. Res.* **2013**, *20*, 3629-3638.

Caliman, F. A.; Gavrilescu, M. *Clean Soil Air Water* **2009**, *37*, 277-303.

Calisto, V.; Esteves, V. I. *Chemosphere* **2009**, *77*, 1257-1274.

Carballa, M.; Fink, G.; Omil, F.; Lema, J. M.; Ternes, T. *Water Res.* **2008**, *42*, 287-295.

Carballa, M.; Omil, F.; Lema, J. M.; Llompart, M.; García-Jares, C.; Rodríguez, I.; Gómez, M.; Ternes, T. *Water Res.* **2004**, *38*, 2918-2926.

Carter, L. J.; Harris, E.; Williams, M.; Ryan, J. J.; Kookana, R. S.; Boxall, A. B. A. *J. Agr. Food Chem.* **2014**, *62*, 816-825.

Carvalho, P. N.; Basto, M. C. P.; Almeida, C. M. R.; Brix, H. *Environ. Sci. Pollut. Res.* **2014**, *21*, 11729-11763.

Celiz, M. D.; Tso, J.; Aga, D. S. *Environ. Toxicol. Chem.* **2009**, *28*, 2473-2484.

Challis, J. K.; Hanson, M. L.; Friesen, K. J.; Wong, C. S. *Environ. Sci. Processes Impacts* **2014**, *16*, 672-696.

Chen, Y.; Zhu, Y.; Wang, Z.; Li, Y.; Wang, L.; Ding, L.; Gao, X.; Ma, Y.; Guo, Y. *Adv. Colloid Interface Sci.* **2011**, *163*, 39-52.

Chenxi, W.; Spongberg, A. L.; Witter, J. D. *Chemosphere* **2008**, *73*, 511-518.

Choi, K.; Kim, Y.; Park, J.; Park, C. K.; Kim, M.; Kim, H. S.; Kim, P. *Sci. Total Environ.* **2008**, *405*, 120-128.

Cincinelli, A.; Martellini, T.; Coppini, E.; Fibbi, D.; Katsoyiannis, A. *Journal of Nanoscience and Nanotechnology* **2015**, *15*, 3333-3347.

Clara, M.; Strenn, B.; Ausserleitner, M.; Kreuzinger, N. *Water Sci. Technol.* **2004a**, *50*, 29.

Clara, M.; Strenn, B.; Kreuzinger, N. *Water Res.* **2004b**, *38*, 947-954.

Clarke, B. O.; Anumol, T.; Barlaz, M.; Snyder, S. A. *Chemosphere* **2015**, *127*, 269-275.

Contardo-Jara, V.; Lorenz, C.; Pflugmacher, S.; Nützmann, G.; Kloas, W.; Wiegand, C. *Aquat. Toxicol.* **2011**, *105*, 428-437.

Cooper, P. F.; Job, G. D.; Green, M. B.; Shutes, R. B. E. *Reed beds and constructed wetlands for wastewater treatment*; WRc Publications: Medmenham, 1996.

de Almeida, C. A. A.; Oliveira, M. S.; Mallmann, C. A.; Martins, A. F. *Environ. Sci. Pollut. Res.* **2015**, *22*, 17192-17201.

De la Cruz, N.; Giménez, J.; Esplugas, S.; Grandjean, D.; de Alencastro, L. F.; Pulgarín, C. *Water Res.* **2012**, *46*, 1947-1957.

De Laurentiis, E.; Chiron, S.; Kouras-Hadef, S.; Richard, C.; Minella, M.; Maurino, V.; Minero, C.; Vione, D. *Environ. Sci. Technol.* **2012**, *46*, 8164-8173.

Deegan, A. M.; Shaik, B.; Nolan, K.; Urell, K.; Oelgemoller, M.; Tobin, J.; Morrissey, A. *Int. J. Environ. Sci. Technol.* **2011**, *8*, 649-666.

Deng, J.; Shao, Y.; Gao, N.; Xia, S.; Tan, C.; Zhou, S.; Hu, X. *Chem. Eng. J.* **2013**, *222*, 150-158.

Derbyshire, F.; Jagtoyen, M.; Andrews, R.; Rao, A.; Martin-Gullon, I.; Grulke, E. A. *Chem. Phys. Carb.* **2001**, *27*, 1-66.

Dietz, A. C.; Schnoor, J. L. *Environ. Health Perspect.* **2001**, *109*, 163-168.

Doll, T. E.; Frimmel, F. H. *Water Res.* **2005**, *39*, 847-854.

Donner, E.; Kosjek, T.; Qualmann, S.; Kusk, K. O.; Heath, E.; Revitt, D. M.; Ledin, A.; Andersen, H. R. *Sci. Total Environ.* **2013**, *443*, 870-876.

Dordio, A. V.; Candeias, A. J. E.; Pinto, A. P.; da Costa, C. T.; Carvalho, A. J. P. *Ecol. Eng.* **2009**, *35*, 290-302.

Dordio, A. V.; Carvalho, A. J. P. *J. Hazard. Mater.* **2013**, *252*□*253*, 272-292.

Dordio, A.; Carvalho, A. J. P.; Teixeira, D. M.; Dias, C. B.; Pinto, A. P. *Bioresour. Technol.* **2010**, *101*, 886-892.

Dordio, A. V.; Gonçalves, P.; Teixeira, D.; Candeias, A. J. E.; Castanheiro, J. E.; Pinto, A. P.; Carvalho, A. J. P. *Intern. J. Environ. Anal. Chem.* **2011**, *91*, 615-631.

Drillia, P.; Stamatelatou, K.; Lyberatos, G. *Chemosphere* **2005**, *60*, 1034-1044.

DrugBank (2017). DrugBank. https://www.drugbank.ca

Du, L. F.; Liu, W. K. *Agron. Sustain. Dev.* **2012**, *32*, 309-327.

Durán-Álvarez, J. C.; Prado, B.; González, D.; Sánchez, Y.; Jiménez-Cisneros, B. *Sci. Total Environ.* **2015**, *538*, 350-362.

Ebele, A. J.; Abou-Elwafa Abdallah, M.; Harrad, S. *Emerging Contam.* **2017**.

Escher, B. I.; Baumgartner, R.; Koller, M.; Treyer, K.; Lienert, J.; McArdell, C. S. *Water Res.* **2011**, *45*, 75-92.

Evgenidou, E. N.; Konstantinou, I. K.; Lambropoulou, D. A. *Sci. Total Environ.* **2015**, *505*, 905-926.

Farré, M. l.; Pérez, S.; Kantiani, L.; Barceló, D. *TrAC Trends Anal. Chem.* **2008**, *27*, 991-1007.

Fatta-Kassinos, D.; Meric, S.; Nikolaou, A. *Anal. Bioanal. Chem.* **2011**, *399*, 251-275.

Fent, K.; Weston, A. A.; Caminada, D. *Aquat. Toxicol.* **2006**, *76*, 122-159.

Ferrari, B.; Paxéus, N.; Giudice, R. L.; Pollio, A.; Garric, J. *Ecotoxicol. Environ. Saf.* **2003**, *55*, 359-370.

Gago-Ferrero, P.; Borova, V.; Dasenaki, M. E.; Thomaidis, N. S. *Anal. Bioanal. Chem.* **2015**, *407*, 4287-4297.

Ganzenko, O.; Huguenot, D.; van Hullebusch, E. D.; Esposito, G.; Oturan, M. A. *Environ. Sci. Pollut. Res.* **2014**, *21*, 8493-8524.

Garcia-Rodriguez, A.; Matamoros, V.; Fontas, C.; Salvado, V. *Environ. Sci. Pollut. Res.* **2014**, *21*, 11708-11728.

García-Santiago, X.; Franco-Uría, A.; Omil, F.; Lema, J. M. *J. Hazard. Mater.* **2016**, *302*, 72-81.

Gavrilescu, M.; Demnerovà, K.; Aamand, J.; Agathos, S.; Fava, F. *New Biotechnol.* **2015**, *32*, 147-156.

Gibson, R.; Durán-Álvarez, J. C.; Estrada, K. L.; Chávez, A.; Jiménez Cisneros, B. *Chemosphere* **2010**, *81*, 1437-1445.

Giri, R. R.; Ozaki, H.; Ota, S.; Takanami, R.; Taniguchi, S. *Int. J. Environ. Sci. Technol.* **2010**, *7*, 251-260.

Göbel, A.; McArdell, C. S.; Joss, A.; Siegrist, H.; Giger, W. *Sci. Total Environ.* **2007**, *372*, 361-371.

Godoy, A. A.; Kummrow, F.; Pamplin, P. A. *Chemosphere* **2015**, *138*, 281-291.

Gomes, R. L.; Scrimshaw, M. D.; Lester, J. N. *Environ. Sci. Technol.* **2009**, *43*, 3612-3618.

Gómez, M. J.; Martínez Bueno, M. J.; Lacorte, S.; Fernández-Alba, A. R.; Agüera, A. *Chemosphere* **2007**, *66*, 993-1002.

González-Pérez, D. M.; Pérez, J. I.; Nieto, M. Á. G. *J. Environ. Sci. Health Part A: Toxic/Hazard. Subst. Environ. Eng.* **2016**, *51*, 855-860.

Gottschall, N.; Topp, E.; Metcalfe, C.; Edwards, M.; Payne, M.; Kleywegt, S.; Russell, P.; Lapen, D. R. *Chemosphere* **2012**, *87*, 194-203.

Gracia-Lor, E.; Ibáñez, M.; Zamora, T.; Sancho, J. V.; Hernández, F. *Environ. Sci. Pollut. Res.* **2014**, *21*, 5496-5510.

Gust, M.; Fortier, M.; Garric, J.; Fournier, M.; Gagné, F. *Sci. Total Environ.* **2013**, *445–446*, 210-218.

Halling-Sørensen, B.; Nors Nielsen, S.; Lanzky, P. F.; Ingerslev, F.; Holten Lützhøft, H. C.; Jørgensen, S. E. *Chemosphere* **1998**, *36*, 357-393.

Hapeshi, E.; Gros, M.; Lopez-Serna, R.; Boleda, M. R.; Ventura, F.; Petrovic, M.; Barceló, D.; Fatta-Kassinos, D. *Clean Soil Air Water* **2015**, *43*, 1272-1278.

Heberer, T. *Toxicol. Lett.* **2002**, *131*, 5-17.

Herklotz, P. A.; Gurung, P.; Vanden Heuvel, B.; Kinney, C. A. *Chemosphere* **2010**, *78*, 1416-1421.

Hijosa-Valsero, M.; Matamoros, V.; Sidrach-Cardona, R.; Martín-Villacorta, J.; Bécares, E.; Bayona, J. M. *Water Res.* **2010**, *44*, 3669-3678.

Hörsing, M.; Ledin, A.; Grabic, R.; Fick, J.; Tysklind, M.; Jansen, J. l. C.; Andersen, H. R. *Water Res.* **2011**, *45*, 4470-4482.

Hua, W.; Bennett, E. R.; Letcher, R. J. *Water Res.* **2006**, *40*, 2259-2266.

Huerta, B.; Rodríguez-Mozaz, S.; Barceló, D. *Anal. Bioanal. Chem.* **2012**, *404*, 2611-2624.

Huerta-Fontela, M.; Galceran, M. T.; Ventura, F. *J. Chromatogr. A* **2010**, *1217*, 4212-4222.

Ikehata, K.; Naghashkar, N. J.; Ei-Din, M. G. *Ozone Sci. Eng.* **2006**, *28*, 353-414.

Im, J. K.; Cho, I. H.; Kim, S. K.; Zoh, K. D. *Desalination* **2012**, *285*, 306-314.

Jarvis, A. L.; Bernot, M. J.; Bernot, R. J. *Sci. Total Environ.* **2014**, *496*, 461-470.

Jekel, M.; Dott, W.; Bergmann, A.; Dünnbier, U.; Gnirß, R.; Haist-Gulde, B.; Hamscher, G.; Letzel, M.; Licha, T.; Lyko, S.; Miehe, U.; Sacher, F.;

Scheurer, M.; Schmidt, C. K.; Reemtsma, T.; Ruhl, A. S. *Chemosphere* **2015**, *125*, 155-167.

Jones, O. A.; Voulvoulis, N.; Lester, J. N. *Water Res.* **2002**, *36*, 5013-5022.

Jones, O. A. H.; Voulvoulis, N.; Lester, J. N. *Crit. Rev. Environ. Sci. Technol.* **2005**, *35*, 401-427.

Joss, A.; Keller, E.; Alder, A. C.; Gobel, A.; McArdell, C. S.; Ternes, T.; Siegrist, H. *Water Res.* **2005**, *39*, 3139-3152.

Joss, A.; Zabczynski, S.; Göbel, A.; Hoffmann, B.; Löffler, D.; McArdell, C. S.; Ternes, T. A.; Thomsen, A.; Siegrist, H. *Water Res.* **2006**, *40*, 1686-1696.

Judd, S. *Trends Biotechnol.* **2008**, *26*, 109-116.

Kadlec, R. H.; Wallace, S. D. *Treatment wetlands*; CRC Press: Boca Raton, 2009.

Kasprzyk-Hordern, B. *Chem. Soc. Rev.* **2010**, *39*, 4466-4503.

Kasprzyk-Hordern, B.; Dinsdale, R. M.; Guwy, A. J. *Water Res.* **2009**, *43*, 363-380.

Katz, B. G.; Griffin, D. W.; Davis, J. H. *Sci. Total Environ.* **2009**, *407*, 2872-2886.

Kim, I.; Yamashita, N.; Tanaka, H. *J. Hazard. Mater.* **2009**, *166*, 1134-1140.

Kim, S. D.; Cho, J.; Kim, I. S.; Vanderford, B. J.; Snyder, S. A. *Water Res.* **2007**, *41*, 1013-1021.

Klamerth, N.; Malato, S.; Maldonado, M. I.; Agüera, A.; Fernández-Alba, A. R. *Environ. Sci. Technol.* **2010**, *44*, 1792-1798.

Klavarioti, M.; Mantzavinos, D.; Kassinos, D. *Environ. Int.* **2009**, *35*, 402-417.

Kleywegt, S.; Pileggi, V.; Yang, P.; Hao, C.; Zhao, X.; Rocks, C.; Thach, S.; Cheung, P.; Whitehead, B. *Sci. Total Environ.* **2011**, *409*, 1481-1488.

König, A.; Weidauer, C.; Seiwert, B.; Reemtsma, T.; Unger, T.; Jekel, M. *Water Res.* **2016**, *101*, 272-280.

Kosjek, T.; Andersen, H. R.; Kompare, B.; Ledin, A.; Heath, E. *Environ. Sci. Technol.* **2009**, *43*, 6256-6261.

Kot-Wasik, A.; Debska, J.; Namiesnik, J. *TrAC Trends Anal. Chem.* **2007**, *26*, 557-568.

Kovalova, L.; Siegrist, H.; Singer, H.; Wittmer, A.; McArdell, C. S. *Environ. Sci. Technol.* **2012**, *46*, 1536-1545.

Kovalova, L.; Siegrist, H.; von Gunten, U.; Eugster, J.; Hagenbuch, M.; Wittmer, A.; Moser, R.; McArdell, C. S. *Environ. Sci. Technol.* **2013**, *47*, 7899-7908.

Kreuzinger, N.; Clara, M.; Strenn, B.; Kroiss, H. *Water Sci. Technol.* **2004**, *50*, 149.

Kruglova, A.; Ahlgren, P.; Korhonen, N.; Rantanen, P.; Mikola, A.; Vahala, R. *Sci. Total Environ.* **2014**, *499*, 394-401.

Kumar, R. R.; Lee, J. T.; Cho, J. Y. *J. Korean Soc. Appl. Biol. Chem.* **2012a**, *55*, 701-709.

Kumar, V.; Johnson, A. C.; Nakada, N.; Yamashita, N.; Tanaka, H. *J. Hazard. Mater.* **2012b**, *227☐228*, 49-54.

Kummerer, K. *J. Environ. Manage.* **2009**, *90*, 2354-2366.

Kümmerer, K. *Pharmaceuticals in the environment: sources, fate, effects and risks*; Springer-Verlag: Berlin, Germany, 2008.

Lajeunesse, A.; Smyth, S. A.; Barclay, K.; Sauvé, S.; Gagnon, C. *Water Res.* **2012**, *46*, 5600-5612.

Lamichhane, K.; Garcia, S. N.; Huggett, D. B.; DeAngelis, D. L.; La Point, T. W. *Arch. Environ. Contam. Toxicol.* **2013**, *64*, 427-438.

Lapworth, D. J.; Baran, N.; Stuart, M. E.; Ward, R. S. *Environ. Pollut.* **2012**, *163*, 287-303.

Larsen, T. A.; Lienert, J.; Joss, A.; Siegrist, H. *J. Biotechnol.* **2004**, *113*, 295-304.

Leclercq, M.; Mathieu, O.; Gomez, E.; Casellas, C.; Fenet, H.; Hillaire-Buys, D. *Arch. Environ. Contam. Toxicol.* **2009**, *56*, 408-415.

Lee, E.; Lee, S.; Park, J.; Kim, Y.; Cho, J. *Drinking Water Eng. Sci.* **2013**, *6*, 89-98.

Lees, K.; Fitzsimons, M.; Snape, J.; Tappin, A.; Comber, S. *Environ. Int.* **2016**, *94*, 712-723.

Li, C.; Cabassud, C.; Guigui, C. *Desalin. Water Treat.* **2014a**, 1-14.

Li, J.; Dodgen, L.; Ye, Q.; Gan, J. *Environ. Sci. Technol.* **2013**, *47*, 3678-3684.

Li, W. C. *Environ. Pollut.* **2014**, *187*, 193-201.

Li, Y. F.; Zhu, G. B.; Ng, W. J.; Tan, S. K. *Sci. Total Environ.* **2014b**, *468*, 908-932.

Li, Z. H.; Zlabek, V.; Velisek, J.; Grabic, R.; Machova, J.; Kolarova, J.; Li, P.; Randak, T. *Ecotoxicol. Environ. Saf.* **2011**, *74*, 319-327.

Lin, W. C.; Chen, H. C.; Ding, W. H. *J. Chromatogr. A* **2005**, *1065*, 279-285.

Lin, Y. C.; Lai, W. W.-P.; Tung, H. h.; Lin, A. Y.-C. *Environ. Monit. Assess.* **2015**, *187*, 256.

Löffler, D.; Römbke, J.; Meller, M.; Ternes, T. A. *Environ. Sci. Technol.* **2005**, *39*, 5209-5218.

López-Serna, R.; Jurado, A.; Vázquez-Suñé, E.; Carrera, J.; Petrovic, M.; Barceló, D. *Environ. Pollut.* **2013**, *174*, 305-315.

Lu, M. C.; Chen, Y. Y.; Chiou, M. R.; Chen, M. Y.; Fan, H. J. *Waste Manage.* **2016**, *55*, 257-264.

Luo, Y.; Guo, W.; Ngo, H. H.; Nghiem, L. D.; Hai, F. I.; Zhang, J.; Liang, S.; Wang, X. C. *Sci. Total Environ.* **2014**, *473□474*, 619-641.

Martin-Diaz, L.; Franzellitti, S.; Buratti, S.; Valbonesi, P.; Capuzzo, A.; Fabbri, E. *Aquat. Toxicol.* **2009**, *94*, 177-185.

Martínez Bueno, M. J.; Agüera, A.; Gómez, M. J.; Hernando, M. D.; García-Reyes, J. F.; Fernández-Alba, A. R. *Anal. Chem.* **2007**, *79*, 9372-9384.

Martucci, A.; Pasti, L.; Marchetti, N.; Cavazzini, A.; Dondi, F.; Alberti, A. *Microporous Mesoporous Mat.* **2012**, *148*, 174-183.

Masoner, J. R.; Kolpin, D. W.; Furlong, E. T.; Cozzarelli, I. M.; Gray, J. L. *Environ. Toxicol. Chem.* **2016**, *35*, 906-918.

Masoner, J. R.; Kolpin, D. W.; Furlong, E. T.; Cozzarelli, I. M.; Gray, J. L.; Schwab, E. A. *Environ. Sci. Processes Impacts* **2014**, *16*, 2335-2354.

Matamoros, V.; Arias, C.; Brix, H.; Bayona, J. *Water Res.* **2009**, *43*, 55-62.

Matamoros, V.; Garcia, J.; Bayona, J. M. *Environ. Sci. Technol.* **2005**, *39*, 5449-5454.

Matamoros, V.; Garcia, J.; Bayona, J. M. *Water Res.* **2008**, *42*, 653-660.

Matamoros, V.; Bayona, J. M. *Environ. Sci. Technol.* **2006**, *40*, 5811-5816.

Matamoros, V.; Puigagut, J.; García, J.; Bayona, J. M. *Chemosphere* **2007**, *69*, 1374-1380.

Maurer, M.; Escher, B. I.; Richle, P.; Schaffner, C.; Alder, A. C. *Water Res.* **2007**, *41*, 1614-1622.

Melin, T.; Jefferson, B.; Bixio, D.; Thoeye, C.; De Wilde, W.; De Koning, J.; van der Graaf, J.; Wintgens, T. *Desalination* **2006**, *187*, 271-282.

Melo-Guimaraes, A.; Torner-Morales, F. J.; Duran-Alvarez, J. C.; Jimenez-Cisneros, B. E. *Water Sci. Technol.* **2013**, *67*, 877-885.

Metcalfe, C. D.; Koenig, B. G.; Bennie, D. T.; Servos, M.; Ternes, T. A.; Hirsch, R. *Environ. Toxicol. Chem.* **2003**, *22*, 2872-2880.

Meyer, W.; Reich, M.; Beier, S.; Behrendt, J.; Gulyas, H.; Otterpohl, R. *Environ. Monit. Assess.* **2016**, *188*, 487.

Meylan, W. M.; Howard, P. H.; Boethling, R. S. *Environ. Toxicol. Chem.* **1996**, *15*, 100-106.

Miao, X. S.; Metcalfe, C. D. *Anal. Chem.* **2003**, *75*, 3731-3738.

Miao, X. S.; Yang, J. J.; Metcalfe, C. D. *Environ. Sci. Technol.* **2005**, *39*, 7469-7475.

Michael, I.; Rizzo, L.; McArdell, C. S.; Manaia, C. M.; Merlin, C.; Schwartz, T.; Dagot, C.; Fatta-Kassinos, D. *Water Res.* **2013**, *47*, 957-995.

Miège, C.; Choubert, J. M.; Ribeiro, L.; Eusèbe, M.; Coquery, M. *Environ. Pollut.* **2009**, *157*, 1721-1726.

Miranda-García, N.; Suárez, S.; Sánchez, B.; Coronado, J. M.; Malato, S.; Maldonado, M. I. *Appl. Catal. B* **2011**, *103*, 294-301.

Mohapatra, D. P.; Brar, S. K.; Tyagi, R. D.; Picard, P.; Surampalli, R. Y. *Sci. Total Environ.* **2013**, *447*, 280-285.

Mohapatra, D. P.; Brar, S. K.; Tyagi, R. D.; Picard, P.; Surampalli, R. Y. *Sci. Total Environ.* **2014**, *470–471*, 58-75.

Mohapatra, D. P.; Cledón, M.; Brar, S. K.; Surampalli, R. Y. *Water Air Soil Pollut.* **2016**, *227*, 77.

Monteiro, S. C.; Boxall, A. B. A. *Rev. Environ. Contam. Toxicol.* **2010**, *202*, 53-154.

Nakada, N.; Shinohara, H.; Murata, A.; Kiri, K.; Managaki, S.; Sato, N.; Takada, H. *Water Res.* **2007**, *41*, 4373-4382.

Nguyen, L. N.; Hai, F. I.; Kang, J. G.; Price, W. E.; Nghiem, L. D. *Int. Biodeterior. Biodegrad.* **2013**, *85*, 474-482.

Nieto, A.; Borrull, F.; Pocurull, E.; Marcó, R. M. *J. Sep. Science* **2007**, *30*, 979-984.

Nieto, A.; Borrull, F.; Pocurull, E.; Marcó, R. M. *Environ. Toxicol. Chem.* **2010**, *29*, 1484-1489.

Noguera-Oviedo, K.; Aga, D. S. *J. Hazard. Mater.* **2016**.

Oetken, M.; Nentwig, G.; Löffler, D.; Ternes, T.; Oehlmann, J. *Arch. Environ. Contam. Toxicol.* **2005**, *49*, 353-361.

Oleszczuk, P.; Pan, B.; Xing, B. *Environ. Sci. Technol.* **2009**, *43*, 9167-9173.

Ort, C.; Lawrence, M. G.; Reungoat, J.; Mueller, J. F. *Environ. Sci. Technol.* **2010**, *44*, 6289-6296.

Pal, A.; Gin, K. Y.-H.; Lin, A. Y.-C.; Reinhard, M. *Sci. Total Environ.* **2010**, *408*, 6062-6069.

Palo, P.; Domínguez, J. R.; Sánchez-Martín, J. *Water Air Soil Pollut.* **2012**, *223*, 5999-6007.

Papageorgiou, M.; Kosma, C.; Lambropoulou, D. *Sci. Total Environ.* **2016**, *543, Part A*, 547-569.

Park, G. Y.; Lee, J. H.; Kim, I. S.; Cho, J. *Water Sci. Technol.* **2004**, *50*, 239-244.

Park, N.; Vanderford, B. J.; Snyder, S. A.; Sarp, S.; Kim, S. D.; Cho, J. *Ecol. Eng.* **2009**, *35*, 418-423.

Paz, A.; Tadmor, G.; Malchi, T.; Blotevogel, J.; Borch, T.; Polubesova, T.; Chefetz, B. *Chemosphere* **2016**, *160*, 22-29.

Pereira, V. J.; Weinberg, H. S.; Linden, K. G.; Singer, P. C. *Environ. Sci. Technol.* **2007**, *41*, 1682-1688.

Petrie, B.; Youdan, J.; Barden, R.; Kasprzyk-Hordern, B. *J. Chromatogr. A* **2016**, *1431*, 64-78.

Petrovic, M.; Barceló, D. *Analysis, fate and removal of pharmaceuticals in the water cycle*; Elsevier: Amsterdam, Netherlands, 2007.

Petrovic, M.; de Alda, M. J. L.; Diaz-Cruz, S.; Postigo, C.; Radjenovic, J.; Gros, M.; Barceló, D. *Philos. Trans. R. Soc. A-Math. Phys. Eng. Sci.* **2009**, *367*, 3979.

Petrovic, M.; Hernando, M. D.; Díaz-Cruz, M. S.; Barceló, D. *J. Chromatogr. A* **2005**, *1067*, 1-14.

Petrovic, M.; Škrbic, B.; Živancev, J.; Ferrando-Climent, L.; Barceló, D. *Sci. Total Environ.* **2014**, *468□469*, 415-428.

Pilon-Smits, E. *Annu. Rev. Plant Biol.* **2005**, *56*, 15-39.

Plumlee, M. H.; Stanford, B. D.; Debroux, J. F.; Hopkins, D. C.; Snyder, S. A. *Ozone Sci. Eng.* **2014**, *36*, 485-495.

Poseidon (2006). Assessment of technologies for the removal of pharmaceuticals and personal care products in sewage and drinking water facilities to improve the indirect potable water reuse (EVK1-CT-2000-00047). Final report. http://poseidon.bafg.de/servlet/is/2888/

Quinn, B.; Gagné, F.; Blaise, C. *Sci. Total Environ.* **2008**, *389*, 306-314.

Rabiet, M.; Togola, A.; Brissaud, F.; Seidel, J. L.; Budzinski, H.; Elbaz-Poulichet, F. *Environ. Sci. Technol.* **2006**, *40*, 5282-5288.

Radjenovic, J.; Jelic, A.; Petrovic, M.; Barceló, D. *Anal. Bioanal. Chem.* **2009**, *393*, 1685-1695.

Radjenovic, J.; Petrovic, M.; Ventura, F.; Barceló, D. *Water Res.* **2008**, *42*, 3601-3610.

Radovic, T.; Grujic, S.; Petkovic, A.; Dimkic, M.; Lauševic, M. *Environ. Monit. Assess.* **2014**, *187*, 4092.

Ramakrishnan, A.; Blaney, L.; Kao, J.; Tyagi, R. D.; Zhang, T. C.; Surampalli, R. Y. *Environ. Earth Sci.* **2015**, *73*, 1357-1368.

Real, F. J.; Benitez, F. J.; Acero, J. L.; Sagasti, J. J. P.; Casas, F. *Ind. Eng. Chem. Res.* **2009**, *48*, 3380-3388.

Reinstorf, F.; Strauch, G.; Schirmer, K.; Gläser, H. R.; Möder, M.; Wennrich, R.; Osenbrück, K.; Schirmer, M. *Environ. Pollut.* **2008**, *152*, 452-460.

Reyes-Contreras, C.; Hijosa-Valsero, M.; Sidrach-Cardona, R.; Bayona, J. M.; Bécares, E. *Chemosphere* **2012**, *88*, 161-167.

Richter, W. J.; Kriemler, P.; Faigle, J. W. *Newer Aspects of the Biotransformation of Carbamazepine: Structural Characterization of Highly Polar Metabolites*; Springer US: Boston, MA, 1978; pp 1-14.

Rivera-Jimenez, S. M.; Lehner, M. M.; Cabrera-Lafaurie, W. A.; Hernández-Maldonado, A. J. *Environ. Eng. Sci.* **2011**, *28*, 171-182.

Rivera-Utrilla, J.; Sánchez-Polo, M.; Ferro-García, M. Á.; Prados-Joya, G.; Ocampo-Pérez, R. *Chemosphere* **2013**, *93*, 1268-1287.

Rizzo, L.; Fiorentino, A.; Grassi, M.; Attanasio, D.; Guida, M. *J. Environ. Chem. Eng.* **2015**, *3*, 122-128.

Robinson, I.; Junqua, G.; Van Coillie, R.; Thomas, O. *Anal. Bioanal. Chem.* **2007**, *387*, 1143-1151.

Rodayan, A.; Majewsky, M.; Yargeau, V. *Sci. Total Environ.* **2014**, *487*, 731-739.

Röhricht, M.; Krisam, J.; Weise, U.; Kraus, U. R.; Düring, R. A. *Clean Soil Air Water* **2009**, *37*, 638-641.

Rosal, R.; Rodríguez., A.; Gonzalo, M. S.; García-Calvo, E. *Appl. Catal. B* **2008**, *84*, 48-57.

Rosario-Ortiz, F. L.; Wert, E. C.; Snyder, S. A. *Water Res.* **2010**, *44*, 1440-1448.

Sabourin, L.; Beck, A.; Duenk, P. W.; Kleywegt, S.; Lapen, D. R.; Li, H.; Metcalfe, C. D.; Payne, M.; Topp, E. *Sci. Total Environ.* **2009**, *407*, 4596-4604.

Sabourin, L.; Duenk, P.; Bonte-Gelok, S.; Payne, M.; Lapen, D. R.; Topp, E. *Sci. Total Environ.* **2012**, *431*, 233-236.

Salgado, R.; Marques, R.; Noronha, J. P.; Carvalho, G.; Oehmen, A.; Reis, M. A. M. *Environ. Sci. Pollut. Res.* **2012**, *19*, 1818-1827.

Santos, J. L.; Aparicio, I.; Callejón, M.; Alonso, E. *J. Hazard. Mater.* **2009**, *164*, 1509-1516.

Santos, L. H. M. L.; Araújo, A. N.; Fachini, A.; Pena, A.; Delerue-Matos, C.; Montenegro, M. C. B. S. *J. Hazard. Mater.* **2010**, *175*, 45-95.

Santos, L. H. M. L.; Gros, M.; Rodriguez-Mozaz, S.; Delerue-Matos, C.; Pena, A.; Barceló, D.; Montenegro, M. C. *Sci. Total Environ.* **2013**, *461*□*462*, 302-316.

Schaider, L. A.; Rudel, R. A.; Ackerman, J. M.; Dunagan, S. C.; Brody, J. G. *Sci. Total Environ.* **2014**, *468–469*, 384-393.

Scheytt, T.; Mersmann, P.; Leidig, M.; Pekdeger, A.; Heberer, T. *Ground Water* **2004**, *42*, 767-773.

Scheytt, T.; Mersmann, P.; Lindstadt, R.; Heberer, T. *Chemosphere* **2005**, *60*, 245-253.

Siegrist, H.; Joss, A. *Water Sci. Technol.* **2012**, *66*, 1369-1376.

Sim, W. J.; Lee, J. W.; Lee, E. S.; Shin, S. K.; Hwang, S. R.; Oh, J. E. *Chemosphere* **2011**, *82*, 179-186.

Simazaki, D.; Kubota, R.; Suzuki, T.; Akiba, M.; Nishimura, T.; Kunikane, S. *Water Res.* **2015**, *76*, 187-200.

Sipma, J.; Osuna, B.; Collado, N.; Monclús, H.; Ferrero, G.; Comas, J.; Rodriguez-Roda, I. *Desalination* **2010**, *250*, 653-659.

Snyder, S. A.; Adham, S.; Redding, A. M.; Cannon, F. S.; DeCarolis, J.; Oppenheimer, J.; Wert, E. C.; Yoon, Y. *Desalination* **2007**, *202*, 156-181.

Spongberg, A. L.; Witter, J. D. *Sci. Total Environ.* **2008**, *397*, 148-157.

Spongberg, A. L.; Witter, J. D.; Acuña, J.; Vargas, J.; Murillo, M.; Umaña, G.; Gómez, E.; Perez, G. *Water Res.* **2011**, *45*, 6709-6717.

SRC (2009). SRC PhysProp Database. http://www.srcinc.com/what-we-do/databaseforms.aspx?id=386

Stackelberg, P. E.; Furlong, E. T.; Meyer, M. T.; Zaugg, S. D.; Henderson, A. K.; Reissman, D. B. *Sci. Total Environ.* **2004**, *329*, 99-113.

Streat, M.; Patrick, J. W.; Perez, M. J. C. *Water Res.* **1995**, *29*, 467-472.

Suarez, S.; Lema, J. M.; Omil, F. *Water Res.* **2010**, *44*, 3214-3224.

Subedi, B.; Balakrishna, K.; Joshua, D. I.; Kannan, K. *Chemosphere* **2017**, *167*, 429-437.

Subedi, B.; Kannan, K. *Sci. Total Environ.* **2015**, *514*, 273-280.

Sui, Q.; Cao, X.; Lu, S.; Zhao, W.; Qiu, Z.; Yu, G. *Emerging Contam.* **2015**, *1*, 14-24.

Sui, Q.; Zhao, W.; Cao, X.; Lu, S.; Qiu, Z.; Gu, X.; Yu, G. *J. Hazard. Mater.* **2017**, *323, Part A*, 99-108.

Sun, J.; Luo, Q.; Wang, D.; Wang, Z. *Ecotoxicol. Environ. Saf.* **2015**, *117*, 132-140.

Sun, S. P.; Zeng, X.; Li, C.; Lemley, A. T. *Chem. Eng. J.* **2014**, *244*, 44-49.

Tadkaew, N.; Hai, F. I.; McDonald, J. A.; Khan, S. J.; Nghiem, L. D. *Water Res.* **2011**, *45*, 2439-2451.

Tahar, A.; Choubert, J. M.; Coquery, M. *Environ. Sci. Pollut. Res.* **2013**, *20*, 5085-5095.

Tahar, A.; Choubert, J. M.; Miège, C.; Esperanza, M.; Le Menach, K.; Budzinski, H.; Wisniewski, C.; Coquery, M. *Environ. Sci. Pollut. Res.* **2014**, *21*, 5660-5668.

Tanoue, R.; Sato, Y.; Motoyama, M.; Nakagawa, S.; Shinohara, R.; Nomiyama, K. *J. Agr. Food Chem.* **2012**, *60*, 10203-10211.

Tchobanoglous, G.; Burton, F. L.; Stensel, H. D.; Metcalf & Eddy *Wastewater engineering: treatment and reuse*; McGraw-Hill Professional, 2003.

Ternes, T.; Loeffler, D.; Knacker, T.; Alder, A. C.; Joss, A.; Siegrist, H. *Abstr. Pap. Am. Chem. Soc.* **2004a**, *228*, U616.

Ternes, T. A. *Water Res.* **1998**, *32*, 3245-3260.

Ternes, T. A.; Joss, A.; Siegrist, H. *Environ. Sci. Technol.* **2004b**, *38*, 392A-399A.

Ternes, T. A.; Kreckel, P.; Mueller, J. *Sci. Total Environ.* **1999**, *225*, 91-99.

Ternes, T. A.; Herrmann, N.; Bonerz, M.; Knacker, T.; Siegrist, H.; Joss, A. *Water Res.* **2004c**, *38*, 4075-4084.

Tixier, C.; Singer, H. P.; Oellers, S.; Muller, S. R. *Environ. Sci. Technol.* **2003**, *37*, 1061-1068.

Tootchi, L.; Seth, R.; Tabe, S.; Yang, P. *Water. Sci. Technol. Water Supply* **2013**, *13*, 1576.

Tran, N. H.; Li, J.; Hu, J.; Ong, S. L. *Environ. Sci. Pollut. Res.* **2014**, *21*, 4727-4740.

Trinh, T.; van den Akker, B.; Stuetz, R. M.; Coleman, H. M.; Le Clech, P.; Khan, S. J. *Water Sci. Technol.* **2012**, *66*, 1856.

Truu, M.; Juhanson, J.; Truu, J. *Sci. Total Environ.* **2009**, *407*, 3958-3971.

Tsao, D. T. *Overview of Phytotechnologies*; Springer Berlin Heidelberg: Berlin, 2003; pp 1-50.

Valdés, M. E.; Amé, M. V.; Bistoni, M. d. l. A.; Wunderlin, D. A. *Sci. Total Environ.* **2014**, *472*, 389-396.

van den Brandhof, E.-J.; Montforts, M. *Ecotoxicol. Environ. Saf.* **2010**, *73*, 1862-1866.

Vedavyasan, C. V. *Desalination* **2000**, *132*, 345-347.

Velagaleti, R. *Drug Inf. J.* **1997**, *31*, 715-722.

Verlicchi, P.; Al Aukidy, M.; Zambello, E. *Sci. Total Environ.* **2012**, *429*, 123-155.

Verlicchi, P.; Al Aukidy, M.; Zambello, E. *Sci. Total Environ.* **2015**, *514*, 467-491.

Verlicchi, P.; Zambello, E. *Sci. Total Environ.* **2015**, *538*, 750-767.

Verlicchi, P.; Zambello, E. *Sci. Total Environ.* **2014**, *470-471*, 1281-1306.

Verliefde, A. R. D.; Cornelissen, E. R.; Heijman, S. G. J.; Verberk, J. Q. J. C.; Amy, G. L.; Van der Bruggen, B.; van Dijk, J. C. *J. Membr. Sci.* **2009**, *339*, 10-20.

Vieno, N.; Tuhkanen, T.; Kronberg, L. *Water Res.* **2007**, *41*, 1001-1012.

Vieno, N. M.; Tuhkanen, T.; Kronberg, L. *J. Chromatogr. A* **2006**, *1134*, 101-111.

Vulliet, E.; Cren-OlivéC.; Grenier-Loustalot, M. F. *Environ. Chem. Lett.* **2011**, *9*, 103-114.

Vymazal, J.; Brix, H.; Cooper, P. F.; Green, M. B.; Haberl, R. *Constructed wetlands for wastewater treatment in Europe*; Backhuys Publishers: Leiden, 1998.

Walters, E.; McClellan, K.; Halden, R. U. *Water Res.* **2010**, *44*, 6011-6020.

Wang, C.; Shi, H.; Adams, C. D.; Gamagedara, S.; Stayton, I.; Timmons, T.; Ma, Y. *Water Res.* **2011**, *45*, 1818-1828.

Wang, J.; Wang, S. *J. Environ. Manage.* **2016**, *182*, 620-640.

Wang, X. H.; Lin, A. Y.-C. *Environ. Pollut.* **2014**, *186*, 203-215.

Wijekoon, K. C.; McDonald, J. A.; Khan, S. J.; Hai, F. I.; Price, W. E.; Nghiem, L. D. *Bioresour. Technol.* **2015**, *189*, 391-398.

Wolf, L.; Zwiener, C.; Zemann, M. *Sci. Total Environ.* **2012**, *430*, 8-19.

Wols, B. A.; Harmsen, D. J. H.; Beerendonk, E. F.; Hofman-Caris, C. H. M. *Chem. Eng. J.* **2014**, *255*, 334-343.

Writer, J. H.; Ferrer, I.; Barber, L. B.; Thurman, E. M. *Sci. Total Environ.* **2013**, *461–462*, 519-527.

Wu, C.; Spongberg, A. L.; Witter, J. D.; Fang, M.; Czajkowski, K. P. *Environ. Sci. Technol.* **2010**, *44*, 6157-6161.

Wu, C.; Spongberg, A. L.; Witter, J. D.; Sridhar, B. B. M. *Ecotoxicol. Environ. Saf.* **2012**, *85*, 104-109.

Wu, X.; Conkle, J. L.; Ernst, F.; Gan, J. *Environ. Sci. Technol.* **2014**, *48*, 11286-11293.

Wu, X.; Dodgen, L. K.; Conkle, J. L.; Gan, J. *Sci. Total Environ.* **2015**, *536*, 655-666.

Yan, Q.; Feng, G.; Gao, X.; Sun, C.; Guo, J. s.; Zhu, Z. *J. Hazard. Mater.* **2016**, *301*, 566-575.

Yangali-Quintanilla, V.; Maeng, S. K.; Fujioka, T.; Kennedy, M.; Li, Z.; Amy, G. *Desalin. Water Treat.* **2011**, *34*, 50-56.

Yoon, Y.; Westerhoff, P.; Snyder, S. A.; Wert, E. C. *J. Membr. Sci.* **2006**, *270*, 88-100.

Yoon, Y.; Westerhoff, P.; Snyder, S. A.; Wert, E. C.; Yoon, J. *Desalination* **2007**, *202*, 16-23.

Yu, Y.; Wu, L. *Talanta* **2012**, *89*, 258-263.

Yu, Z.; Peldszus, S.; Huck, P. M. *Water Res.* **2008**, *42*, 2873-2882.

Yuan, S.; Jiang, X.; Xia, X.; Zhang, H.; Zheng, S. *Chemosphere* **2013**, *90*, 2520-2525.

Zenker, A.; Cicero, M. R.; Prestinaci, F.; Bottoni, P.; Carere, M. *J. Environ. Manage.* **2014**, *133*, 378-387.

Zhang, D. Q.; Gersberg, R. M.; Ng, W. J.; Tan, S. K. *Environ. Pollut.* **2014**, *184*, 620-639.

Zhang, D. Q.; Tan, S. K.; Gersberg, R. M.; Sadreddini, S.; Zhu, J. F.; Nguyen, A. T. *Ecol. Eng.* **2011**, *37*, 460-464.

Zhang, D. Q.; Gersberg, R. M.; Zhu, J.; Hua, T.; Jinadasa, K. B. S. N.; Tan, S. K. *Environ. Pollut.* **2012**, *167*, 124-131.

Zhang, W.; Ding, Y.; Boyd, S. A.; Teppen, B. J.; Li, H. *Chemosphere* **2010**, *81*, 954-960.

Zhang, Y.; Geißen, S. U.; Gal, C. *Chemosphere* **2008**, *73*, 1151-1161.

Zhao, X.; Metcalfe, C. D. *Anal. Chem.* **2008**, *80*, 2010-2017.

Zhou, H.; Smith, D. W. *Can. J. Civ. Eng.* **2001**, *28*, 49-66.

Zorita, S.; Martensson, L.; Mathiasson, L. *Sci. Total Environ.* **2009**, *407*, 2760-2770.

In: Carbamazepine
Editor: Bernadette A. Woods

ISBN: 978-1-53611-954-1
© 2017 Nova Science Publishers, Inc.

Chapter 4

THE EVALUATION OF DIFFERENT REACTOR CONFIGURATIONS IMMOBILIZED WITH *PHANEROCHAETE CHRYSOSPORIUM* ON THE LONG-TERM CARBAMAZEPINE REMOVAL FROM NON-STERILE SYNTHETIC WASTEWATER

Xueqing Li[1,2], Wai Chi Lau[1], Renata Alves de Toledo[1] and Hojae Shim[1,*]

[1]Department of Civil and Environmental Engineering, Faculty of Science and Technology, University of Macau, Macau SAR, China
[2]Water Environmental Research Institute, Shenzhen Academy of Environmental Science, Shenzhen, China

ABSTRACT

Carbamazepine (CBZ) is a pharmaceutically active compound that has been detected in many water bodies worldwide and is classified as a micropollutant. CBZ is hardly biodegraded (removal efficiency <10%) through the conventional activated sludge process and the white-rot

---

* Corresponding author: Hojae Shim. Department of Civil and Environmental Engineering, Faculty of Science and Technology, University of Macau, Macau SAR, China. Email: hjshim@umac.mo.

fungus (WRF) is reported the only microorganism to degrade it efficiently. Even though the WRF reactor has been applied to remove CBZ from wastewater, the performances varied considerably. In addition, it is still difficult to maintain a stable long-term reactor performance due to the bacterial contamination. This study aims to enhance the removal performance of WRF reactor toward CBZ under non-sterile conditions during long-term operation. The possibility of a WRF strain *Phanerochaete chrysosporium* immobilized on wooden chips to remove CBZ under non-sterile conditions was investigated. The CBZ removal efficiency in artificially contaminated water was improved around 30% in 7 days when the fungal immobilization was used. Adsorption was the main contributor to the CBZ removal at the early stage. However, bioremoval was considered the main removal mechanism afterwards. A countercurrent seepage bioreactor with *P. chrysosporium* immobilized on wooden chips was developed and continuously fed with synthetic domestic wastewater spiked with CBZ (1,000 µg/L) under non-sterile conditions for 165 days. The average removal efficiency for CBZ reached 78.28 ± 5.77%. The countercurrent seepage mode bioreactor proved to be conducive to increase the fungal resistance to the contamination by indigenous bacteria. The performance of CBZ removal was also evaluated under different reactor configuration consisted of a rotating suspension cartridge reactor immobilized with *P. chrysosporium* on polyurethane foam cubes. The reactor was continuously operated under non-sterile conditions for 160 days. The removal efficiency for CBZ exceeded 90% after one month of fungal adaptation by applying the intermittent operation mode and the progressive cut of external carbon source feeding. The CBZ removal mainly occurred biologically and adsorption accounted for only 7.7%. The bacterial contamination was suppressed effectively under non-sterile conditions for both reactor configurations considered as promising alternatives for the CBZ treatment in contaminated water.

Keywords: bacterial contamination, carbamazepine, non-sterile condition, reactor configuration, white rot-fungus

INTRODUCTION

The pharmaceutically active compounds (PhACs), ingredients of personal care products, hormones, and other chemicals, are reported frequently detected in sewage and sewage-impacted surface waters. Many of them are suspected to have an adverse impact on humans and wildlife. The water reuse practices, therefore, raise concern due to the potential adverse health effects associated with these wastewater derived PhACs. Most of them are of the anthropogenic origin, and due to their incomplete elimination during wastewater treatment, the sewage treatment plant effluents are their important discharge points to the receiving water bodies. For over a century, the conventional activated sludge (CAS) process has been widely used for both municipal and industrial wastewater treatments. However, CAS has not been designed with the aim of PhACs removal. As a result, more advanced treatment techniques for the removal of PhACs from water and wastewater such as advanced oxidation, activated carbon adsorption, membrane filtration, advanced biological processes, or combined hybrid process have been proposed. Nonetheless, none of them has shown the removal solution due to the lack of applicability to a wide range of PhACs.

White-rot fungus (WRF) shows a high capability to oxidize different types of recalcitrant contaminants including polycyclic aromatic hydrocarbons (PAHs), synthetic dyes, and polychlorinated biphenyls (PCBs) (Bosso and Cristinzio, 2014; Cruz-Morato et al., 2013; Field and Serra-Alvarez, 2008; Haritash and Kaushik, 2009; Khan et al., 2013). The possibility to apply WRF to the PhACs removal from wastewater has also been evaluated due to the non-specific nature of WRF oxidative enzymes, including laccase, peroxidases, and cytochrome P450 (Demarche et al., 2012; Jelic et al., 2012; Nguyen et al., 2014; Zhang and Geißen, 2010). Considering the most important step in developing the WRF technology is the design of a suitable bioreactor, the reactor configurations developed so far include fluidized bed bioreactor, packed bed bioreactor, stirred tank bioreactor, trickle-bed bioreactor, membrane bioreactor, and rotating biological contactor (Cruz-Morato et al., 2013; Jelic et al., 2012; Nguyen et al., 2013; Novotny et al., 2012; Pakshirajan and Kheria, 2012; Rodarte-Morales et al., 2012; Yang et al., 2013b). The respective PhACs were almost completely removed using those configurations but most reactors were operated under sterile conditions. Only very few studies were carried out continuously under non-sterile conditions.

A membrane bioreactor (MBR) inoculated with a WRF *Trametes versicolor* was applied to continuously remove a mixture of bisphenol A and diclofenac in synthetic wastewater under non-sterile conditions (Yang et al., 2013a). The removal performances for both micropollutants were lower, compared to the ones obtained in batch tests using pure fungal cultures. The lower removal performance in the continuous mode was associated with bacterial contamination and enzyme loss. The same behavior was also observed by the study of Nguyen et al. (2013), where the continuous removal of 30 micropollutants in an MBR containing a mixed culture of WRF and bacteria significantly dropped, compared to the results obtained in batch test. In general, regardless of the micropolluntant type, a drop in the removal performance would follow when the reactor was operated continuously under non-sterile conditions. The reactor performance deterioration is attributed to the bacterial overgrowth which further inhibits fungal growth and enzyme production to some extent (Yang et al., 2013a; Zhou et al., 2013). Therefore, the inhibition of bacterial growth is important during the WRF long-term reactor operation by creating an environment where fungi can dominate over bacteria.

The utilization of different types of immobilization techniques in WRF systems has received a considerable attention in recent years. The advantages of microbial immobilization include protection of microbial cells from shear damage, favorable mass transfer and oxygen supply, reduction of protease activity and contamination risk, and more resistance to the environmental perturbations (pH variation and toxic chemicals) (Couto, 2009). Many works have been developed to immobilize enzymes as biocatalysts to remove PhACs (Nair et al., 2013; Songulashvili et al., 2012). The immobilization of single enzymes has a limited application considering different classes/nature of PhACs as well as their complex separation and purification steps. Therefore, the whole-cell immobilized WRF is favorable (Yang et al., 2013a) but only a few studies on the PhACs removal utilize it. The objective of current work is to explore the removal mechanisms for carbamazepine, as the target PhAC, by the WRF immobilization when different reactor configuration strategies were applied for the long-term operation under non-sterile conditions.

MATERIALS AND METHODS

Microorganism

Phanerochaete chrysosporium strain BKM-F-1767 (obtained from the Guangdong Institute of Microbiology, China) was stored at -18°C until used. The modified PDA medium was used to collect the fungal spores and consisted of (per liter) 3 g KH_2PO_4, 20 g agar, 20 g glucose, 8 mg thiamin, 1.5 g $MgSO_4 \cdot 7H_2O$ with 20% potato extract. *P. chrysosporium* strain was inoculated onto the PDA plates and incubated for 10 days at 30°C. Sterile distilled water was used to rinse the white spores from the PDA plates, resulting in a spore suspension of ~14.0 × 10^6 spores/mL. The spore suspension was then stored at 4°C until used.

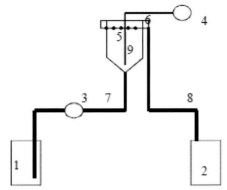

1. Influent tank. 2. Effluent tank. 3. Feed pump. 4. Air pump. 5. Reactor. 6. Steel mesh.
   7. Inlet pipe. 8. Outlet pipe. 9. Diffuser.

Figure 1. Schematic of WRF fixed-bed reactor.

Chemicals

Carbamazepine ($C_{15}H_{12}N_2O$) was purchased from the Sigma-Aldrich (US). The stock solution (1.0 g/L) was prepared in methanol and stored at 4°C. All the other chemicals used were of analytical grades.

Synthetic Wastewater

The synthetic wastewater (enzyme-producing medium) was prepared following Kirk et al. (1978). The medium was prepared in 1 L tap water and contained 2 g glucose, 0.66 g ammonium tartrate, 1 g KH_2PO_4, 0.5 g $MgSO_4·7H_2O$, 0.1 g $CaCl_2·2H_2O$, 1 mg thiamine, and 1 mL Tween 80. The pH was adjusted to 4.5 with 50 mM sodium tartrate buffer.

Carriers

Wooden Chips

Cunninghamia is one of the main tree species in southern China and its wooden chips (10-20 mm length x 5-10 mm width x 0.2 mm thickness) were used as the carrier materials for fungal immobilization.

Polyurethane Foam Cubes

The polyurethane foam cubes ($1.0 \times 1.0 \times 1.0$ cm^3; density, 74 kg/m^3) were also used as matrices for fungal immobilization. The polyurethane foam is considered an excellent support for the microbial immobilization due to its stability and mechanical strength.

Reactor Set-Up and Operation

Fixed-bed bioreactor

The reactor (3 L working volume) was made of methyl methacrylate with a lower inverted conical (6 cm height, 4.5 cm diameter at the bottom) and an upper cylinder (14 cm height, 16 cm diameter) (Figure 1). Wastewater was fed and discharged from bottom and top, respectively. The mixture of *P. chrysosporium* mycelia pellets and wooden chips were filled inside the reactor. Details about the preparation of fungal mycelia and wooden chips can be found elsewhere (Li et al., 2015a). Aeration was supplied by an air pump (Aquarium Air Pump, Hailea Co., Ltd, China) to maintain the dissolved oxygen (DO) concentration at ≥ 4 mg/L. The effects of 8.25% sodium hypochlorite addition and hydrolytic retention time (HRT) on carbamazepine removal performance were evaluated. By adjusting pump flow and feeding interval, three HRT levels (0.6, 19, and 65 h) were studied. In the later part of the reactor operation, 8.25% sodium hypochlorite was added twice into the influent (1:100, v/v).

Countercurrent Seepage Bioreactor

The bioreactor (3 L working volume; Figure 2) was made of methyl methacrylate (70 cm height, 7.5 cm diameter). The synthetic wastewater was fed from the top at a flow rate of 10 mL/min. Details about the reactor operation can be found elsewhere (Li et al., 2015b). The flakes exhibited cardhouse fabric, after packed into the reactor with porosity and specific area of 90% and 103 cm^2/cm^3, respectively. The porosity (n) was calculated as follows.

$$n = \frac{V_v}{V} = \frac{V - V_w}{V}; \; V_w = \frac{W_w}{\gamma_w} \tag{1}$$

where V_v is the void volume (cm³), V is the reactor volume (cm³), V_w is the total volume of the flakes inside the reactor (cm³), W_w is the air-dried weight of the flakes (kg), and γw is the air-dried density of the flakes (kg/m³).

The bioreactor was continuously operated under non-sterile conditions for 165 days. The reactor was fed with synthetic wastewater spiked with 1,000 μg/L carbamazepine. Ammonium tartrate was fed (0.2 g/L) during the whole operational period while the glucose load was gradually reduced in stages, at 10, 5, 2.5, and 0.5 g/L during day 0 to 20, day 21 to 67, day 68 to 148, and after day 149, respectively. No biomass was supplemented or discharged from the bioreactor during the whole operational period.

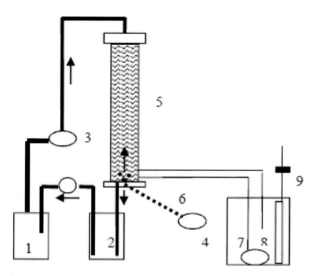

1. Influent tank. 2. Effluent tank. 3. Feed pump. 4. Air pump. 5. Reactor. 6. Air supply. 7. Submerged pump. 8. Heater. 9. Temperature controller.

Figure 2. Schematic of countercurrent seepage bioreactor.

Rotating Suspension Cartridge Reactor

Twelve stainless steel mesh cartridges (3.5 cm x 6.0 cm x 4.0 cm) were allocated on a stainless disk (diameter, 14 cm) inside the reactor. The cartridges were filled with polyurethane foam cubes (1.0 x 1.0 x 1.0 cm³) immobilized with *P. chrysosporium*. Details about the reactor operation can be found elsewhere (Li et al., 2016). The glucose concentration in the synthetic wastewater fed into the reactor was 10 g/L before day 74 and was further cut to 5 (day 74), 2.5 (day 94), and 1.0 g/L (day 118). The reactor HRT was 3 days by controlling feed and effluent pumps (Figure 3). No biomass was replenished or wasted from the reactor during its continuous operation.

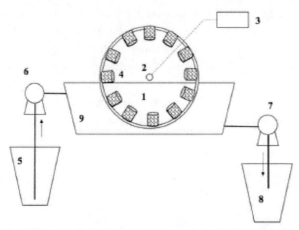

1. Rotating disk. 2. Electric shaft. 3. Intermittent switch. 4. Cartridges. 5. Influent tank. 6. Feed pump. 7. Effluent pump. 8. Storage tank. 9. Reaction tank.

Figure 3. Schematic of rotating suspension cartridge reactor.

Removal Mechanism Study in WRF Immobilized System

Comparison Test for Free Growing and Immobilized WRF Systems

Around 1.0 g/L wooden chips (~0.5 mm) were added to 150 mL synthetic wastewater in flask under non-sterile condition. The control flask did not contain wooden chips but only synthetic wastewater instead. Both flasks were inoculated with the WRF spore suspension (1:50, v/v) and shaken at 90 rpm for one week. Schematic of countercurrent seepage bioreactor. C and 90 rpm for one week. After this period, carbamazepine was spiked into both flasks at 20 mg/L. A mixed liquid sample was taken daily from each flask during 7 days and then centrifuged (5430R centrifuge, Eppendorf, Germany) for 30 min at 7,830 rpm. The carbamazepine concentration and the activities of the two major extracellular enzymes (lignin peroxidase, LiP and manganese peroxidase, MnP) were measured from the supernatant, and the biomass dry weight was measured from the pellets.

Wooden Chips Adsorption Test

Different amounts of wooden chips (1, 5, 10, 15, and 20 g/L) were added into each flask with synthetic wastewater (50 mL) and carbamazepine (10 mg/L), and the flasks were incubated at 30°C and 90 rpm. The residual carbamazepine concentration was measured in every 30 min until reached the adsorption equilibrium.

Biomass Adsorption Test

The *P. chrysosporium* spore suspension (1:50, v/v) was inoculated into a potato dextrose liquid medium (without agar) and incubated at 30°C. A mycelia layer (thickness 0.3-1.0 cm) was formed after 5 days at the air-liquid interface. It was aseptically separated from the liquid medium and autoclaved at 121°C (20 min). The inactivated biomass was also used in the adsorption test following the same procedure described in the wooden chips adsorption test.

Rotating Suspension Cartridge Reactor Study

Carrier Dimension Comparison

The polyurethane foam cubes (3 g) with different dimensions (5.0 × 3.5 × 2.5 cm^3 and 1.0 × 1.0 × 1.0 cm^3) were added into flasks containing the culture medium (200 mL). The flasks were then autoclaved at 121°C for 20 min. The WRF spore suspension was inoculated (1:40, v/v) into the flasks at room temperature and incubated at 30°C and 100 rpm. After one week, both flasks were spiked with carbamazepine (1,000 μg/L). The extracellular enzyme activities were then measured after 4 and 7 days.

Carbamazepine Removal Mechanism

The polyurethane foam cubes (1.0 × 1.0 × 1.0 cm^3) were added into flasks containing 100 mL culture medium, followed by sterilization, WRF spore suspension addition, and incubation. After 5 days of incubation, one flask was sterilized and set as control. Carbamazepine was spiked (1,000 μg/L) into both flasks and samples were taken after 12 h, 1, 2, and 3 days, to measure the carbamazepine residual concentration.

Carbamazepine Removal in a Co-Existing System with Indigenous Microorganisms

A dominant strain of indigenous microorganisms that contaminated the reactor was isolated from the mixed liquid at the end of reactor operation. The detailed information about the respective microbial identification can be found elsewhere (Li et al., 2016). The bacterial isolate showed the highest homology with *Bacillus sphaericus* (accession number DQ286312.1). A liquid culture medium containing (per liter) 10 g peptone, 5 g beef extract, and 5 g NaCl (pH 7.2-7.4) was used to inoculate the isolate to prepare the respective bacterial suspension. Six flasks containing 250 mL synthetic wastewater were autoclaved and inoculated with suspensions of *P. chrysosporium* and *B. sphaericus* at the same ratio (1:40, v/v), followed by the incubation at 25°C and 250 rpm for five days. Each flask was then spiked with different carbamazepine concentrations (400, 800, 1,000, 4,000, 7,000, and 10,000 µg/L). The carbamazepine residual concentration and the biomass dry weight were measured for each flask after 24 hours. Five tubes containing 5 mL solution of different glucose concentrations (2.5, 10, 20, 30 and 40 g/L) and 0.2 g/L ammonia tartrate were also autoclaved and then spiked with 1,000 µg/L carbamazepine. The suspensions of *P. chrysosporium* and *B. sphaericus* were inoculated at 1:40 (v/v) into each tube. All the inoculated tubes were incubated at 25°C and 120 rpm. The residual concentrations of carbamazepine and the biomass dry weight for each were measured after 24 hours.

Analytical Assays

Dionex UltiMate 3000 HPLC-Diode array detector system (Thermo Scientific, US) equipped with Acclaim™ C30 column (5 µm, 4.6 x 150 mm) was used to measure carbamazepine concentrations with the injection volume of 100 µL. The details about the HPLC operational conditions for the carbamazepine analysis can be found elsewhere (Li et al., 2015b).

The activities of lignin peroxidase (LiP) and manganese peroxidase (MnP) were measured following the Dye Azure B assay described by Archibald (1992) and by Aitken and Irvine (1989), respectively. The total nitrogen (TN) and the chemical oxygen demand (COD) were measured by the standard HACH methods. The dissolved oxygen (DO) concentrations and the pH values were measured using Orion™ Star A323 (Thermo Scientific, US) and S220 SevenCompact™ (Mettler-Toledo Group, Switzerland), respectively.

The supernatants used for the bacterial and fungal plate counting were obtained from the mixed liquid samples taken from the bioreactor and centrifuged at 7,830 rpm and 30°C. The standard method for the spread plating technique was from Eaton and Franson (2005). The culture medium for bacteria consisted of 10 g peptone, 5 g beef extract, 5 g NaCl, and 20 g agar per one liter of distilled water (pH 7.2-7.4). WRF was cultivated in PDA medium plates. Both microorganisms were incubated at their optimal temperatures (WRF, 30°C and bacteria, room temperature). After two days, the colonies formed were counted in colony forming units (CFU/mL).

The mixed liquid taken from the WRF system was filtered through glass microfiber filters (1.0 μm, Whatman, Schleicher and Schuell). The retentate and the filtrate which represented the biomass dry weight of *P. chrysosporium* and bacterial isolate, respectively, were dried in an oven (80°C) until no changes in weight were observed.

Statistical Analysis

The statistical analysis was carried out by using the software SPSS. Data for the carbamazepine removal efficiencies in two different cultivation types (suspension and immobilization), the extracellular enzyme activity, and the carbamazepine removal efficiency in two different carrier sizes (1.0 x 1.0 x 1.0 cm^3 and 5.0 x 3.5 x 2.5 cm^3) as well as the carbamazepine removal efficiency when the reactor was operated in mode I (5 min running/15 min stop) and mode II (5 min running/5 min stop) were statistically analyzed by one-way analysis of variance (ANOVA) at 95% confidence (p = 0.05). All the experiments were conducted in triplicates and repeated independently to ensure a high level of confidence for the experimental data.

RESULTS AND DISCUSSION

Free Growing vs. Immobilized Systems

After 7 days of incubation, approximately 13 mg/L carbamazepine (originally added at 20 mg/L) were still remained in the free growing system under non-sterile conditions, with the removal efficiency of 34 ± 2.15%. In comparison, the removal efficiency reached 61.30 ± 3.84% when WRF was immobilized on wooden chips, 28% higher than the free growing system. A better dye decolorization efficiency was also obtained when WRF was immobilized on plastic tubes (Hai et al., 2013). Gao et al. (2008) also observed a high level of enzyme activity when WRF was immobilized under non-sterile conditions, attributed to the higher resistance of WRF to the bacterial proliferation.

In general, the carbamazepine removal efficiency was much higher during the first 24 hours compared to the 7-day removal. The extracellular enzymes (LiP and MnP) were monitored daily (Figure 4) and at 24 hours after the carbamazepine addition, a sharp decline of the MnP activity was observed (4,150 to 730 U/L) while the LiP activity remained low (370-490 U/L) compared to its average level (621 U/L) during the whole experimental period. These results suggest both enzymes were not associated with the substantial carbamazepine removal during the first 24 hours. Subsequently, to further understand the carbamazepine removal mechanism, the adsorption and removal by crude enzymes were carried out.

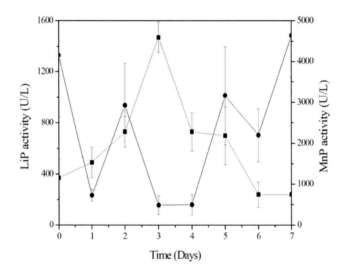

Figure 4. Variation of two main extracellular enzymes activity: LiP (−■−) and MnP (−●−), produced by the immobilized *P. chrysosporium* during the batch experimental period.

Adsorption by Wooden Chips and Biomass

The adsorption capacities of the adsorbents are mainly determined through the adsorption isotherm study, and the carbamazepine removal was determined through the variation between the initial and final concentrations during the reaction period. Table 1 shows the adsorption process for the carbamazepine removal on wooden chips fitted better to the Langmuir isotherm model than the Freundlich model. The carbamazepine sorption capacity (q_{max}) at 30°C was 0.06 mg/g, suggesting the compound does not have high affinity to adsorb on the wooden chips surface and the removal observed was mainly due to the biological process. The obtained results are also in accordance with Nguyen et al. (2014), showing the adsorption without a substantial removal of carbamazepine (only 6%). The low adsorption capacity of carbamazepine could be attributed to its low log K_{ow} (2.45), characteristics of hydrophilic compounds (log K_{ow} values ≤ 3) and usually subjected to the limited sorption (Yang et al., 2013a). The results show adsorption played a major role within 24 hours but the biological removal was the main mechanism for the carbamazepine removal.

Removal by Crude Enzyme

The residual carbamazepine concentration did not change within the crude enzyme test period. Zhang and Geißen (2012) also reported the carbamazepine removal efficiency was not that substantial (<10%) in the presence of LiP produced by *P. chrysosporium*, further suggesting the carbamazepine removal may be more dependent on the WRF intracellular enzyme system instead. The importance of cytochrome P450 in carbamazepine degradation has been reported in many studies (Marco-Urrea et al., 2009; Nguyen et al., 2014; Zhang and Geißen, 2012).

Table 1. Adsorption capacities of wooden chips and inactivated biomass for carbamazepine for Langmuir and Freundlich isotherm models

Adsorbent	Langmuir model			Freundlich model		
	q_{max} (mg/g)	b (L/mg)	R^2	K_f	n^{-1}	R^2
Wooden chips	0.06	1.17	0.86	0.03	0.56	0.79
Inactivated biomass	0.01	0.91	0.57	0.08	14.28	0.81

q_{max} (mg/g) is the maximum adsorption capacity; b (L/mg) is the Langmuir adsorption constant, related to the adsorption energy.

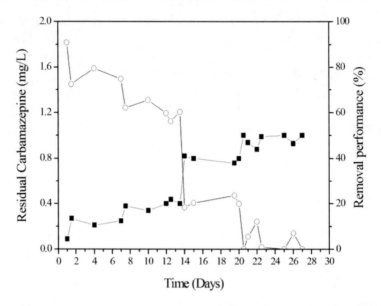

Figure 5. Carbamazepine removal (residual concentration: —■—; removal efficiency: —○—) over time.

Fixed-Bed Bioreactor

A fixed-bed reactor (Figure 1) was applied to study the carbamazepine removal performance by the immobilized *P. chrysosporium* under the non-sterile continuous operation for 4 weeks. The effect of HRT on carbamazepine removal and the potential inhibitory effect of bacterial contamination in the reactor were also evaluated through the selective disinfection (8.25% sodium hypochlorite added at 1:100).

Carbamazepine was removed within two weeks (removal efficiencies, 60-80%). When the HRT was prolonged to 65 hours on day 4 and day 10, even though the carbamazepine removal increased slightly (with 3.5% and 7% higher removal efficiencies, respectively, than the previous ones), the overall removal trend decreased. A sharp decline of the removal efficiency (from 60% to 20%) was observed on day 14, which is associated with the bacterial contamination. Both types of microorganisms would compete for nutrients and substrates, limiting the fungal growth to some extent (Gao et al., 2008). Despite the disinfectant (sodium hypochlorite) addition on day 20 and day 25, the carbamazepine removal efficiencies dropped even further (Figure 5). Even though the activities of extracellular enzymes generated by *P. chrysosporium* were recovered by the sodium hypochlorite addition (Li et al., 2015a), its addition did not affect the fungal intracellular enzyme system which is crucial for the biological removal of carbamazepine.

Sankaran et al. (2010) considered the importance to apply a moderate bactericidal dose that could inhibit the bacterial growth without suppressing the fungal cell growth and enzyme production. Zhou et al. (2013) further stated the addition of ozone as a bactericide in the WRF system suppressed the bacterial contamination without a negative impact on the fungal activities. On the other hand, sodium hypochlorite used in current study is an oxidant capable of oxidizing many recalcitrant xenobiotic compounds by transforming into the equivalent biodegradable forms. Therefore, it would also be possible sodium hypochlorite was associated in the carbamazepine removal. Additional studies are still necessary to better evaluate the application of different types of bactericides and their effects on the WRF system.

Countercurrent Seepage Bioreactor

The countercurrent reactor was designed to reproduce the WRF natural habitat. WRF is commonly found in the forest ecosystems on moist stumps (Singh and Singh, 2014). WRF colonized rot the stumps by forming a biofilm on the wooden surface. The suitable living conditions for WRF and its ability to resist to the bacterial proliferation are established by exposing the biofilm to atmosphere and to the rainwater flowing down to its surface. To mimic this situation, the reactor was filled up with wooden flakes immobilized with *P. chrysosporium*. The synthetic wastewater was fed from top to bottom, and according to the resistance generated from the wooden flakes, the flow rates were adjusted accordingly. The wastewater moved slowly along the flake surface forming a thin layer, favoring the contact between the *P. chrysosporium* growing on the flakes and the wastewater. The air was supplied from bottom to top. Another cylindrical reactor with the equivalent working volume (3 L; 15 cm height, 16 cm diameter) was operated in a concurrent submerged mode (i.e., both wastewater and air were supplied into the reactor from the bottom and discharged from the top) in parallel with the countercurrent seepage bioreactor during the first four weeks. The DO levels in both operational modes were monitored, and different flows of synthetic wastewater (5, 10, 23, and 45 mL/min) with the fixed glucose loading (2.5 g/L) were evaluated in terms of carbamazepine removal and enzyme activity.

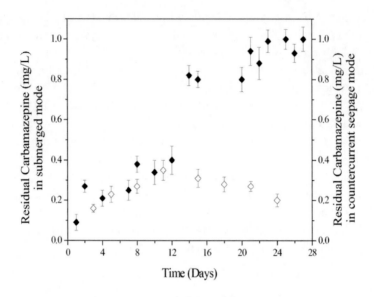

Figure 6. Carbamazepine removal in the submerged mode (—◆—) and the countercurrent seepage mode (—◇—) reactors over time.

Around 60-80% carbamazepine were removed in the first two weeks and a sharp drop in the removal efficiency (<20%) was observed in the submerged reactor after day 14 (Figure 6). As discussed above, this reactor deterioration may be associated with the bacterial contamination (Zhou et al., 2013). In comparison, however, this drop in the carbamazepine removal efficiency was not observed in the countercurrent seepage bioreactor. Two bioreactors have different dimensions but the same working volume (3 L), suggesting the wastewater has the same contact time with the microorganisms in both reactors. Considering the same other experimental conditions (pH, temperature, HRT, and wastewater loading rate) were applied to both reactors, different flow patterns inside the reactors were critical to keep the reactor operation stable without the bacterial contamination.

Even though air was supplied in both reactors at the same flow rate (6.50 L/min), the DO level measured in the countercurrent seepage mode (8.5 mg/L) was about 20% higher compared to the submerged mode (6.8 mg/L). It is well known oxygen plays a vital role in *P. chrysosporium* degradation activity and physiological metabolism. The association between *P. chrysosporium* growth, glucose consumption, and lignin decomposition was evaluated when the fungal cultures were in contact with different oxygen concentrations (5%, 21%, and 100%) (Kirk et al., 1978). Regardless of the oxygen concentration,

P. chrysosporium growth was similar within three days of incubation with 25% glucose consumed in current study. The lignin mineralization to carbon dioxide initiated in flasks containing 21% and 100% oxygen after the initial growth period, occurring three times faster in 100% oxygen compared to 21%. Even though Leisola et al. (1983) stated the oxygen limitation was the primary reason for the incomplete lignin degradation by *P. chrysosporium* in non-agitated cultures, in current study, it was considered the oxygen concentration not that important and the oxygen transfer or its diffusion inside the cell more important instead. There are some advantages in the application of countercurrent seepage mode instead of submerged mode in the oxygen migration from air to liquid. First, the countercurrent flow generates a shearing action on the gas-liquid interface, favorable for the oxygen migration. Secondly, a relatively longer flow path is created by the flakes in cardhouse, which favors oxygen diffusion from the bubbles to the liquid.

The influence of the flow rate on the bioreactor treatment performance was evaluated to better understand the countercurrent seepage mode characteristics. The removal efficiency for carbamazepine slightly decreased (82.57 ± 2.37% to 81.36 ± 1.42%) and the MnP activity dropped (1.75 ± 0.32 U/L to 0.95 ± 0.27 U/L) when the feeding flow was varied from 5 to 45 mL/min (Figure 7). The results are in agreement with the ones obtained by Hai et al. (2013) where the enzyme activity dropped significantly when the HRT was reduced from 4.5 days to 1 day in a WRF-MBR continuously operated under non-sterile conditions. The attenuation on enzyme activity was attributed to the enzyme washout under short HRT conditions. In current work, the efficient oxygen transfer and the low flow rate applied in the countercurrent seepage mode protect the fungal activity and the respective enzyme production to some extent, inhibiting the bacterial contamination effectively.

Carbamazepine Removal

The reactor was operated continuously (Figure 8) and a stable carbamazepine removal (nearly 80%) was obtained during 165 days. Carbamazepine is known by its recalcitrant nature and WRF is reported the only microorganism capable of degrading it but the removal efficiencies reported are not that substantial. The WRF technology has been applied to the carbamazepine removal from wastewater (Cruz-Morato et al., 2013; Jelic et al., 2012; Nguyen et al., 2013; Rodarte-Morales et al., 2012) but the removal performances varied from more than 50% removal (Rodarte-Morales et al., 2012; Zhang and Geißen, 2012) to almost no removal (Cruz-Morato et al., 2013). The results obtained in current study are promising to remove carbamazepine under non-sterile conditions, showing the best performance in removing this well-known recalcitrant compound using a bioreactor continuously operated.

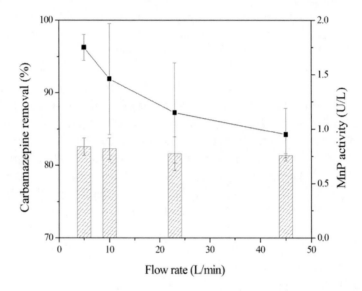

Figure 7. Effect of the flow rate on carbamazepine removal efficiency (▨) and MnP activity (—■—) in the countercurrent seepage bioreactor.

To further assess the role of glucose addition to the influent feed in the carbamazepine removal, experiments were carried out using deionized waster spiked with carbamazepine (1.0 g/L) and inoculated with *P. chrysosporium* spore suspension. The flask was incubated for one week, and during this period there was no obvious fungal growth and the concentration of carbamazepine kept stable, in agreement with Kirk et al. (1976) who reported the important role of external carbon source in *P. chrysosporium* growth and proved the fungus would neither grow nor degrade other substrate if carbamazepine were the only carbon source available in the culture medium. Other growth substrate (glucose or cellulose) might be present because the low energy generated by the lignin degradation would support the fungal growth (Kirk et al., 1976). Other studies also reported the importance of other carbon source to support the fungal growth to improve the WRF treatment performance. Pakshirajan and Kheria (2012) stated a 30% improvement in the decolorization rate was obtained when 5 g/L glucose was supplemented into a textile wastewater treatment process using immobilized *P. chrysosporium.* Novotny et al. (2012) also suggested the decolorization of dyes was associated with the glucose consumption and when the glucose concentration was low (1 mM), the decolorization stopped. On the other hand, the corresponding average removal efficiencies for carbamazepine were 73, 79, 80, and 73% when the glucose load was reduced in the feed, from the initial 10 g/L to 5, 2.5, and 0.5 g/L on day 21, day 68, and day 149, respectively (Figure 8). A slight decline in the removal efficiencies was observed on day 149 when the feed glucose concentration became as low as 0.5 g/L. This decrease could be attributed to the proteases generated by *P. chrysosporium* under glucose-limited conditions, which are responsible for the decay of WRF enzymes (mainly LiP) (Blanquez et al., 2008). It should also be noted this decline in the reactor performance occurred during the later operational period (day 149), still suggesting a good stability of this bioreactor to remove carbamazepine.

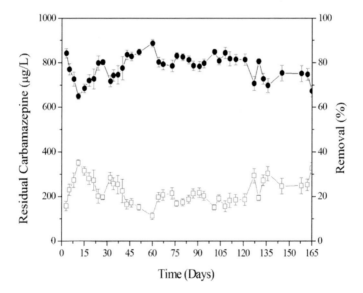

Figure 8. Carbamazepine removal efficiencies using the countercurrent seepage bioreactor (—●—) and its residual concentrations (—□—) over 165 days.

Effects of pH, Bacterial Contamination, and MnP Activity

The effluent pH fluctuated around 4.0 at the early stage of reactor operation probably due to the acidogenic bacteria activities under glucose-sufficient conditions (Cruz-Morato et al., 2013). The pH increased when the glucose load in the feed sharply declined after day 67 and this increase was associated with the inhibition of both aerobic and acidogenic bioactivities (Zhang and Geißen, 2012). On day 94, pH reached 6.0 and then remained stable until day 134 but decreased to 4.0 on day 135 (Figure 9).

The number of bacterial colonies inside the bioreactor remained stable (<0.2 x 10^6 CFUs/mL) while the fungal colonies tended to decrease gradually (from 0.6 x 10^6 CFUs/mL to 0.2 x 10^6 CFUs/mL) in 20 days and undetectable after day 148 (Figure 10). The results are in agreement with Yang et al. (2013b), reporting the bacterial contamination in the bioreactor would disturb the fungal growth considerably. The bacterial contamination occurred in the bioreactor was successfully inhibited throughout the whole operational period, shown by the stable level of bacterial colonies observed.

The MnP activity was detected at a relatively low level (less than 3.0 U/L), and the result is similar to other studies dealing with WRF reactors operated under non-sterile conditions (Gao et al., 2008; Hai et al., 2012; Yang et al., 2013b; Zhang and Geißen, 2012). The low LiP activity may be related to the bacterial contamination, which would have an inhibition effect on the *P. chrysosporium* enzyme production (Zhang and Geißen, 2012).

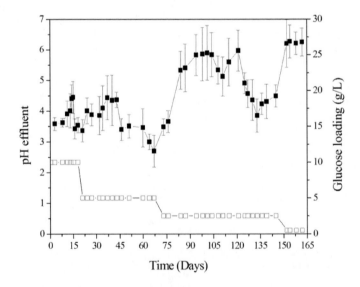

Figure 9. Variations in feed glucose loading (—□—) and effluent pH (—■—) in countercurrent seepage bioreactor over time.

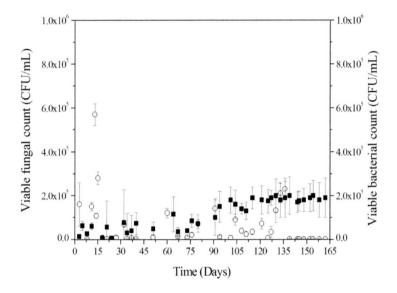

Figure 10. Viable fungal (—○—) and bacterial (—■—) counts in effluent.

The effectiveness on bacterial suppression was a result of different strategies applied to the bioreactor. The WRF immobilization is known to enhance enzyme production (Gao et al., 2008) and the utilization of wooden chips in current study favors fungal growth since the carrier can also be used as growth substrate for fungi in nature. Temperature is an important operational parameter in the reactor (Jin et al., 1999) and was controlled (30°C) to support the WRF growth over bacteria. The effluent pH values were around 6, also favorable in suppressing the bacterial growth. In addition, the gradual decrease of influent glucose feeding was also favorable to WRF growth and bacterial suppression.

Rotating Suspension Cartridge Reactor

Optimization of the Operational Conditions

Carrier Size

Figure 11 shows that the removal efficiency for carbamazepine and the activity of the extracellular enzyme produced by *P. chrysosporium* are higher in the system with $1.0 \times 1.0 \times 1.0$ cm^3 (6.00 cm^2/cm^3) polyurethane foam cubes as carriers compared to $5.0 \times 3.5 \times 2.5$ cm^3 (1.77 cm^2/ cm^3) cubes. There are statistically significant differences (p) between the extracellular enzyme production (0.009) as well as the carbamazepine removal efficiency (0.0037) and the different carrier sizes. The carriers with the larger specific surface area have more sites to immobilize the fungal cells, yielding higher production of enzymes and better removal performances. The smaller carrier size would also bring some disadvantages since the narrow passage resulting from the small space between the carriers' aggregate would make difficult for fungi to extend their mycelia on the small carrier surface (even making the fungal mycelium to be wrapped and overlapping), thus reducing the contact area between fungus and liquid/air.

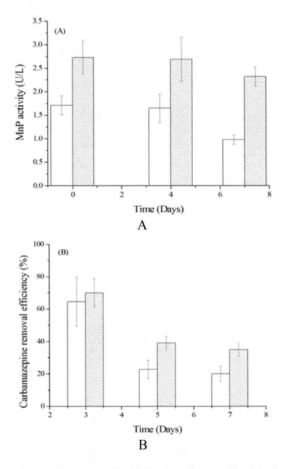

Figure 11. Comparison of (A) extracellular enzyme (MnP) activity and (B) carbamazepine removal efficiency in *P. chrysosporium* systems immobilized on 5.0 × 3.5 × 2.5 cm^3 (□) and 1.0 × 1.0 × 1.0 cm^3 (▨) polyurethane foam cubes.

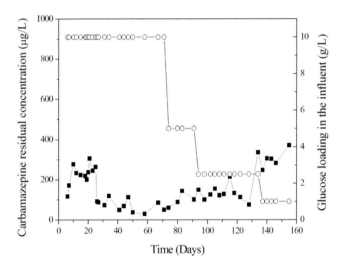

Figure 12. The residual concentrations of carbamazepine (-■-) in the effluent and the glucose loading (-○-) in the influent.

Run/Stop Cycle

The removal efficiency for carbamazepine achieved under 5 min run/15 min stop (mode II) was approximately 20% higher compared to 5 min run/5 min stop (mode I; average removal efficiency, 71%). There are statistically significant differences in carbamazepine removal efficiency (0.0024) between modes I and II. The longer stop time brought more contact opportunities between WRF and oxygen in the air. It is also well known that the lignin degradation is an oxidative process which has a high O_2 requirement (Leisola et al., 1983).

Carbamazepine Removal

Based on the optimization study, $1.0 \times 1.0 \times 1.0$ cm^3 polyurethane foam cubes were used as the carriers filled into the bioreactor cartridges with the run/stop time of 5 min/15 min during the continuous operation. Although carbamazepine has usually been detected at the level of ng/L to µg/L in the environment, the concentration as high as mg/L was also found in some cases such as the effluent from a pharmaceutical industry (Lester et al., 2013). In the current study, 1,000 µg/L of carbamazepine was selected to evaluate the effectiveness of the fungal reactor in degrading this compound. After one month of adaptation, the carbamazepine removal efficiency was higher than 90% (day 31-74; as high as $91.34 \pm 5.77\%$) (Figure 12). Compared to other previous studies, the removal performance obtained in this study confirms the operational mode of run/stop cycle favored a better bioreactor treatment performance while the polyurethane foam cubes inside the cartridge provided high porosity and promoted air and liquid circulation. The gradual cut of carbon source loading in the influent also contributed to the carbamazepine removal to some extent (Li et al., 2016).

No control experiments (without inoculated fungus) were carried out during 160 days to evaluate the contribution of indigenous microorganisms to carbamazepine removal. Instead, some shake flasks experiments were carried out, spiked with carbamazepine at 1,000 µg/L. The removal efficiency for carbamazepine in the inoculated system was around 35%. Almost no carbamazepine removal (<5%) was observed in the control with indigenous microorganisms only, which suggests the non-specific enzyme system of *P. chrysosporium* has an important role in the carbamazepine removal.

Enzyme Activity and Bacterial Contamination

The activity of the extracellular enzyme remained at a relatively low level during the whole operational period. The MnP activity detected was always no more than 3.5 U/L, indicating carbamazepine was degraded even under the peroxidase-suppressing conditions (Li et al., 2016). The low enzyme activity has also been observed when the continuous WRF reactor was operated under non-sterile conditions. Sima et al. (2012) reported MnP and laccase activities were always less than 2.2 and 5.0 U/L, respectively, in a rotating drum biological contactor using *Irpex lacteus* for treating textile wastewater. Rodarte-Morales et al. (2012) also found the MnP activity detected below 30 U/L for a fixed-bed reactor immobilized with *P. chrysosporium* to remove some PhACs including carbamazepine. Zhang and Geißen (2012) reported LiP occasionally detected at a very low activity while MnP not detected in a plate bioreactor immobilized with *P. chrysosporium*, applied to degrade carbamazepine. In comparison, there have been very few studies reporting the relatively high enzyme activity. Pakshirajan and Kheria (2012) reported the MnP activity ranged from 400 to 2,000 U/L while the LiP activity was no more than 300 U/L in a rotating biological contactor (RBC) reactor using *P. chrysosporim* to treat textile wastewater. The bacterial counting also showed the growth of viable bacteria has continuously been inhibited to below 2.0×10^6 CFUs/mL during the whole operational period (Figure 10), which proved the bacterial overgrowth inside the bioreactor suppressed effectively.

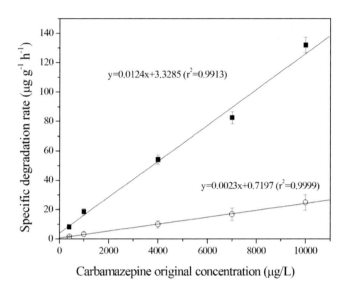

Figure 13. The specific degradation rates of *P. chrysosporium* (-■-) and *B. sphaericus* (-○-) in a coexisting system.

Removal Mechanism for Carbamazepine

The contribution of physical and biological processes to the carbamazepine removal (1,000 μg/L) was evaluated using polyurethane foam cubes immobilized with *P. chrysosporium*. After 3 days, carbamazepine remained at 790.46 ± 30.21 μg/L and 983.89 ± 48.13 μg/L in the active and autoclaved systems, respectively. The adsorption accounted for less than 10% (~7.7%) of the total removal. The result is also consistent with other studies. Rodarte-Morales et al. (2012) applied the polyurethane foam immobilized with *P. chrysosporium* in a fixed-bed reactor to remove some PhACs including carbamazepine and showed the residual concentrations of PhACs on the polyurethane foam support quite low (the residual carbamazepine was 1.43 mg/g polyurethane foam). The biosorption process also showed a limited contribution in other previous studies for the carbamazepine removal (Daughton and Ternes, 1999; Luo et al., 2014). Therefore, the main mechanism for the carbamazepine removal in current system is considered the biological removal instead of adsorption.

Carbamazepine Removal in Co-Existing System

Figure 13 shows the specific degradation rates of both types of microorganisms increased nearly linearly, proportional to the original carbamazepine concentrations. The average specific degradation rate of *P. chrysosporium* was about 4.4 times higher compared to *B. sphaericus*. When the glucose loading in matrix enhanced from 2.5 to 10 g/L, the specific degradation rate of *P. chrysosporium* dropped from 0.98 ± 0.41 to 0.53 ± 0.29 μg/g·h and became stabilized until the glucose loading reached 20 g/L (Figure 14). A similar trend was found for *B. sphaericus*, showing the specific degradation rate for carbamazepine almost reduced linearly when the glucose loading in matrix increased (i.e., 2.79 ± 0.35, 1.81 ± 0.42, and 0.80 ± 0.33 μg/g·h of specific degradation rates corresponding to 2.5, 10, and 20 g/L glucose loading) and tends to slow down when the glucose load was higher than 30 g/L (Figure 14).

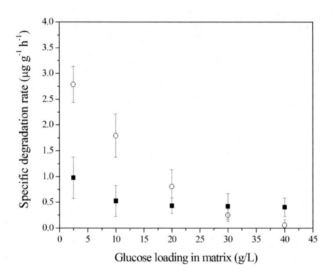

Figure 14. Effect of carbon source loading on the specific degrading rates of *P. chrysosporium* (-■-) and *B. sphaericus* (-○-) in a coexisting system.

CONCLUSION

Two different WRF reactors (countercurrent seepage bioreactor and rotating suspension cartridge reactor) were established to effectively remove carbamazepine as a recalcitrant pharmaceutical compound from the synthetic wastewater during a stable long-term operation under non-sterile conditions. The countercurrent seepage bioreactor immobilized with *P. chrysosporium* was stably operated for almost half a year under non-sterile conditions, with the removal efficiency for carbamazepine of about 80%. The countercurrent seepage mode contributes to increase the WRF resistance to the bacterial contamination occurring in the bioreactor. The rotating suspension cartridge reactor immobilized with *P. chrysosporium* on the polyurethane foam cubes was continuously operated for about 160 days to remove carbamazepine from the synthetic wastewater under non-sterile conditions. The removal efficiency higher than 90% was achieved under the optimized conditions of 1.0 x 1.0 x 1.0 cm^3 sized polyurethane foam cubes used as carriers, 10 g/L glucose added to the influent as the external carbon source, and 5 min run/15 min stop cycle used as the operational mode. The biological (fungal) removal was the main mechanism for carbamazepine removal in these fungal bioreactors. The developed process could be used as an advanced treatment unit for further removing the recalcitrant chemicals from the wastewater treatment plants effluents.

ACKNOWLEDGMENTS

This research was supported by the University of Macau Multi-Year Research Grant (MYRG2014-00112-FST) and by grants from the Macau Science and Technology Development Fund (FDCT/061/2013/A2 and FDCT/063/2013/A2).

REFERENCES

Aitken, M., Irvine, R., 1989. Stability testing of ligninase and Mn-peroxidase from *Phanerochaete chrysosporium*. *Biotechnol. Bioeng.* 34, 1251-1260.

Archibald, F., 1992. A New Assay for Lignin-Type Peroxidases Employing the Dye Azure B. *Appl. Environ. Microbiol.* 58, 3110-3116.

Blánquez, P., Sarràand, M., Vicent, T., 2008. Development of a continuous process to adapt the textile wastewater treatment by fungi to industrial conditions. *Process Biochem.* 43, 1-7.

Bosso, L., Cristinzio, G., 2014. A comprehensive overview of bacteria and fungi used for pentachlorophenol biodegradation. *Rev. Environ. Sci. Biotechnol.* 13, 387-427.

Couto, S., 2009. Dye removal by immobilised fungi. *Biotechnol. Adv.* 27, 227-235.

Cruz-Morato, C., Ferrando-Climent, L., Rodriguez-Mozaz, S., Barcelo, D., Marco-Urrea, E., Vicent, T., Sarra, M., 2013. Degradation of pharmaceuticals in non-sterile urban wastewater by *Trametes versicolor* in a fluidized bed bioreactor. *Water Res.* 47, 5200-5210.

Daughton, C., Ternes, T., 1999. Pharmaceuticals and personal care products in the environment: Agents of subtle change? *Environ. Health Perspect.* 107, 907-938.

Demarche, P., Junghanns, C., Nair, R., Agathos, S., 2012. Harnessing the power of enzymes for environmental stewardship. *Biotechnol. Adv.* 30, 933-953.

Eaton, A., Franson, A., 2005. *Standard methods for the examination of water and wastewater.* Washington, D.C., American Public Health Association.

Field, J., Serra-Alvarez, R., 2008. Microbial transformation and degradation of polychlorinaed biphenyls. *Environ. Pollut.* 155, 11-12.

Gao, D., Zeng, Y., Wen, X., Qian, Y., 2008. Competition strategies for the incubation of white rot fungi under non-sterile conditions. *Process Biochem.* 43, 937-944.

Hai, F., Yamamoto, K., Nakajimac, F., Fukushi, K., 2012. Application of a GAC-coated hollow fiber module to couple enzymatic degradation of dye on membrane to whole cell biodegradation within a membrane bioreactor. *J. Membrane Sci.* 389, 67-75.

Hai, F., Yamamoto, K., Nakajima, F., Fukushi, K., Nghiem, L., Price, W., Jin, B., 2013. Degradation of azo dye acid orange 7 in a membrane bioreactor by pellets and attached growth of *Coriolus versicolour*. *Bioresour. Technol.* 141, 29-34.

Haritash, A., Kaushik, C., 2009. Biodegradation aspects of polycyclic aromatic hydrocarbons (PAHs): A review. *J. Hazard. Mater.* 169, 11-15.

Jelic, A., Cruz-Morato, C., Marco-Urrea, E., Sarra, M., Perez, S., Vicent, T., Petrovic, M., Barcelo, D., 2012. Degradation of carbamazepine by *Trametes versicolor* in an air pulsed fluidized bed bioreactor and identification of intermediates. *Water Res.* 46, 955-964.

Jin, B., van Leeuwen, H., Patel, B., Doelle, H., Yu, Q., 1999. Production of fungal protein and glucoamylase by *Rbizopus oligosporus* from starch processing wastewater. *Process Biochem.* 34, 59-65.

Khan, R., Bhawana, P., Fulekar, M., 2013. Microbial decolorization and degradation of synthetic dyes: A review. *Rev. Environ. Sci. Biotechnol.* 12, 75-97.

Kirk, T., Connors, W., Zeikus, J., 1976. Requirement for a growth substrate during lignin decomposition by two wood-rotting fungi, *Appl. Environ. Microbiol.* 32, 192-194.

Kirk, T., Schultz, E., Connors, W., Lorenz, L., Zeikus, J., 1978. Influence of culture parameters on lignin metabolism by *Phanerochaete chrysosporium. Arch. Microbiol.* 117, 277-285.

Leisola, M., Ulmer, D., Fiechter, A., 1983. Problem of oxygen transfer during degradation of lignin by *Phanerochaete chrysosporium. Eur. J. Appl. Microbiol. Biotechnol.* 17(2), 113-116.

Lester, Y., Mamane, H., Zucker, I., Avisar, D., 2013. Treating wastewater from a pharmaceutical formulation facility by biological process and ozone. *Water Res.* 47, 4349-4356.

Li, X., de Toledo, R.A., Wang, S., Shim, H., 2015a. Removal of carbamazepine and naproxen by immobilized *Phanerochaete chrysosporium* under non-sterile condition. *New Biotechnol.* 32, 282-289.

Li, X., Xu, J., de Toledo, R.A., Shim, H., 2015b. Enhanced removal of naproxen and carbamazepine from wastewater using a novel countercurrent seepage bioreactor immobilized with *Phanerochaete chrysosporium* under non-sterile conditions. *Bioresour. Technol.* 197, 465-474.

Li, X., Xu, J., de Toledo, R.A., Shim, H., 2016. Enhanced carbamazepine removal by immobilized *Phanerochaete chrysosporium* in a novel rotating suspension cartridge reactor under non-sterile condition. *Int. Biodeter. Biodegr.* 115, 102-109.

Luo, Y., Guo, W., Ngo, H., Nghiem, L., Hai, F., Zhang, J., Liang, S., Wang, X., 2014. A review on the occurrence of micropollutants in the aquatic environment and their fate and removal during wastewater treatment. *Sci. Total Environ.* 473-474, 619-641.

Marco-Urrea, E., Perez-Trujillo, M., Vicent, T., Caminal, G., 2009. Ability of white-rot fungi to remove selected pharmaceuticals and identification of degradation products of ibuprofen by *Trametes versicolor. Chemosphere* 74, 765-772.

Nair, R., Demarche, P., Agathos, S., 2013. Formulation and characterization of an immobilized laccase biocatalyst and its application to eliminate organic micropollutants in wastewater. *New Biotechnol.* 30, 814-823.

Nguyen, L., Hai, F., Yang, S., Kang, J., Leusch, F., Roddick, F., Price, W., Nghiem, L., 2013. Removal of trace organic contaminants by an MBR comprising a mixed culture of bacteria and white-rot fungi, *Bioresour. Technol.* 148, 234-241.

Nguyen, L., Hai, F., Yang, S., Kang, J., Leusch, F., Roddick, F., Price, W., Nghiem, L., 2014. Removal of pharmaceuticals, steroid hormones, phytoestrogens, UV-filters, industrial chemicals and pesticides by *Trametes versicolor*: Role of biosorption and biodegradation. *Int. Biodeter. Biodegr.* 88, 169-175.

Novotný, C., Trošt, N., Šlušla, M., Svobodová, K., Miesková, H., Válková, H., Malachová, K., Pavko, A., 2012. The use of the fungus *Dichomitus squalens* for degradation in rotating biological contactor conditions. *Bioresour. Technol.* 114, 241-246.

Pakshirajan, K., Kheria, S., 2012. Continuous treatment of coloured industry wastewater using immobilized *Phanerochaete chrysosporium* in a rotating biological contactor reactor. *J. Environ. Manage.* 101, 118-123.

Rodarte-Morales, A., Feijoo, G., Teresa Moreira, M., Juan, M., 2012. Evaluation of two operational regimes: fed-batch and continuous for the removal of pharmaceuticals in a fungal stirred tank reactor. *Chem. Eng. Trans.* 27, 151-156.

Sankaran, S., Khanal, S., Jasti, N., Jin, B., Pometto, A., van Leeuwen, J., 2010. Use of Filamentous Fungi for Wastewater Treatment and Production of High Value Fungal Byproducts: A Review. *Crit. Rev. Environ. Sci. Technol.* 40, 400-449.

Sima, J., Pocedic, J., Roubickova, T., Hasal, P., 2012. Rotating Drum Biological Contactor and its Application for Textile Dyes Decolorization. *Procedia Eng.* 42, 1579-1586.

Singh, A., Singh, T., 2014. Biotechnological applications of wood-rotting fungi: A review. *Biomass Bioenerg.* 62, 198-206.

Songulashvili, G., Jimenez-Tobon, G., Jaspers, C., Penninckx, M.J., 2012. Immobilized laccase of *Cerrena unicolor* for elimination of endocrine disruptor micropollutants. *Fungal Biol.* 116, 883-889.

Yang, S., Hai, F., Nghiem, L., Price, W., Roddick, F., Moreira, M., Magram, S., 2013a. Understanding the factors controlling the removal of trace organic contaminants by white-rot fungi and their lignin modifying enzymes: A critical review. *Bioresour. Technol.* 141, 97-108.

Yang, S., Hai, F., Nghiem, L., Nguyen, L., Roddick, F., Price, W., 2013b. Removal of bisphenol A and diclofenac by a novel fungal membrane bioreactor operated under non-sterile conditions. *Int. Biodeter. Biodegr.* 85, 483-490.

Zhang, Y., Geißen, S.U., 2010. In vitro degradation of carbamazepine and diclofenac by crude lignin peroxidase. *J. Hazard. Mater.* 176, 1089-1092.

Zhang, Y., Geiβen, S.U., 2012. Elimination of carbamazepine in a non-sterile fungal bioreactor. *Bioresour. Technol.* 112, 221-227.

Zhou, C., Wen, X., Ning, P., 2013. Continuous Acid Blue 45 decolorization by using a novel open fungal reactor system with ozone as the bactericide. *Biochem. Eng. J.* 79, 246-252.

INDEX